HEALTH PROMOTION IN IRELAND

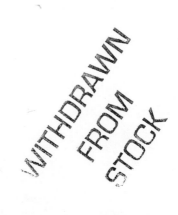

HEALTH PROMOTION IN IRELAND

*Denis Ryan, Patricia Mannix McNamara
and Christine Deasy*

GILL & MACMILLAN

Gill & Macmillan
Hume Avenue
Park West
Dublin 12
with associated companies throughout the world
www.gillmacmillan.ie

ISBN-13: 978 0 7171 4024 4
ISBN-10: 0 7171 4024 5

Index compiled by Cover to Cover
Print origination in Ireland by O'K Graphic Design, Dublin

The paper used in this book is made from the wood pulp of managed forests. For every tree felled, at least one is planted, thereby renewing natural resources.

A catalogue record is available for this book from the British Library.

Contents

Preface   vi

Acknowledgments   vii

Introduction   ix

Section 1: Health Promotion Theory and Principles

Chapter 1: The Nature of Health and Health Promotion   1

Chapter 2: Health Promotion and Public Policy   21

Chapter 3: Health Promotion and Change Management   34

Chapter 4: Health Promotion and Empowerment   48

Chapter 5: Health Promotion, Lifestyle Issues and Work   55

Chapter 6: Issues and Themes in Health-promotion Practice   73

Section 2: Research and Health Promotion

Chapter 7: Evidence-based Practice   103

Chapter 8: Research Paradigms   108

Chapter 9: Critical Theory   113

Chapter 10: Phenomenology   116

Chapter 11: Grounded Theory   123

Chapter 12: Action Research   126

Chapter 13: Evaluation   133

Chapter 14: Ethics and Health-promotion Research   139

Chapter 15: Conducting Literature Reviews   146

Chapter 16: Interviews   151

Chapter 17: Focus Groups   157

Chapter 18: Surveys   165

Chapter 19: Writing Your Research Proposal   173

References   178

Index   199

Preface

Health Promotion in Ireland is a text that reflects the conceptual frameworks underpinning health promotion but does so from a uniquely Irish perspective. This edition also reflects our belief and commitment to the values that underpin health promotion as deeply important. We believe the values of empowerment, advocacy and partnership should permeate all work in health promotion, be it conceptual, pragmatic or both.

The book is presented in two sections. Section 1 outlines health-promotion theory and principles and offers critiques specific to Irish policy and practice. Section 2 explores research paradigms and methods that are commensurate with the values and practice of health promotion. As evidence-based practice is important to the development of any profession we believe that developing the capacity of health-promotion practitioners in research is the first step to support them in generating their own evidence of good practice.

Acknowledgments

We would like to acknowledge the support and patience of our families as we devoted much time not only to writing but also to debating the concepts we include in this text. This meant much sacrificing of time with loved ones and we appreciate the patience and generosity of their giving up of that time without complaint. Particularly thanks to Ann, Julianne, Aisling, Stephen, Mike, Barry and Conor. Finally our thanks to friends and colleagues in the Department of Nursing and Midwifery and the Department of Education and Professional Studies, University of Limerick.

Introduction

Health promotion as a distinct area of interest, theory and practice can be dated to the 1980s. While it is still a relatively new concept, the principles underpinning health promotion are not new. Health promotion is not, or should not be, the preserve of health professionals exclusively. Believing that it is demonstrates a fundamental misunderstanding of health promotion. However this is an unfortunate though fairly widely held misapprehension.

Health promotion is underpinned by a specific ideology and espouses a set of values and beliefs. In particular health promotion is driven by a commitment to the promotion of *health for all* as a central premise. Therefore the values of health promotion dictate that health promotion is not reactive in nature but rather is proactive in the promotion of the awareness of the centrality of health in people's lives. The value of justice is implicit in the most influential literatures of health promotion. The Ottawa Charter (World Health Organization, 1986), which still remains the cornerstone upon which most if not all health-promotion initiatives are based, indicates the importance of advocacy as key to the success of health promotion. Advocacy in support of those who cannot articulate their needs, and particularly in supporting individuals and communities in developing their own advocacy skills, is central to such health-promotion endeavours as community development. Empowerment is also at the heart of health promotion. It is the foundation for the types of relationships that health practitioners need to develop with their clients, be they individuals or communities. When the Ottawa Charter defines health promotion as 'the process of enabling people to increase control over and improve their health' (WHO, 1986:2) it is clear that both advocacy and empowerment are the hub around which all else is built.

Placing such justice-based values as advocacy and empowerment at the heart of health promotion means that client centredness becomes integral to health-promotion practice – as it should be. These are not simple concepts. To place empowerment at the centre of health-promotion practice means that the professional practice itself becomes a new landscape. For many who have comfortably worked within the medical model (where the expert holds autonomy and power), placing the voice of the client in equal partnership in the process of the promotion of their health is a deep challenge. Indeed for clients who have previously experienced a medical model only, the challenge is as great. It requires a letting go of traditional understandings of what it means to be practitioner and client. Equally, it means the taking on of new and paradoxically more liberating processes of working. When the client takes on more responsibility for engaging in attitudinal or behavioural change, the practitioner then must adopt the role of facilitator and guide. Supporting advocacy for clients requires courage and commitment on the part of practitioners. Supporting advocacy may be popular among the clients or communities. However it may not be so popular with groups who may be challenged by the process and/or outcome of advocacy, such as professional or other parties with vested interests.

Building healthy public policy is a key function of health promotion. Health promotion and public health are very closely allied. Effective health-promotion initiatives can and should increase public health. Heath promotion as an enterprise and as a driving force in policy formation and practice delivery is driven by principles of holism and is client centred. In health promotion, health is seen as a resource rather than an end in its own right. It is understood as an approach that has application across a broad range of professional practice areas. Health promotion is not limited to any single professional group, but should underpin the practice of anyone dealing with health or human services where there is a relationship with health status.

Health-promotion practitioners are influenced by a wide range of theoretical perspectives which inform their thinking and guide their practice. It is precisely this openness to draw from relevant theories from many disciplines that makes health promotion adaptive and is one of its greatest strengths. Health promotion draws on established theories and models from areas such as psychology and sociology as well as other social and biological sciences and the humanities. It does so to explore holistic explanations for human behaviour at individual and group levels as well as perspectives on health and health promotion.

Health promotion acts as a unifying force between individual, group and community-level interventions and broader societal interests and influences. It does so at a sociopolitical level in terms of influencing and contributing to policy formulation. It is involved at a structural and community level through programme development and implementation with groups. Programme development places the needs of groups and communities at the heart of its work, therefore client centredness is a prerequisite. Needs assessment and evaluation processes become integral to health promotion. Needs assessment is an important tool in supporting groups and communities to articulate their needs. A normative approach is not commensurate with health-promotion practice. Evaluation is key to evidencing good practice in health promotion but more importantly, it gives the community or groups the opportunity to assess the efficacy and suitability of health-promotion initiatives.

The health-promotion practitioner does not operate in a vacuum. They are influenced by relevant theory. The role of theory and its integration with practice is an obvious prerequisite for successful health promotion. Theory remains a sterile entity if it fails to be implemented and reviewed or developed. Therefore the health-promotion agent requires the ability to learn the theory, apply it in practice and evaluate the process and the application of knowledge.

This book has been guided by these themes and concerns. It is structured in such a way that it introduces the reader to the key theoretical discourses and research in health promotion. Therefore it is divided into two sections. Section 1 reflects the theoretical basis of health promotion and the application and evaluation of practice. Section 2 considers research paradigms and practice that we consider pertinent to health promotion.

Chapter 1 explores the competing interests and influences on the definition of health. This chapter discusses the domains of influence on health and health status, otherwise referred to in literature as health determinants. A discussion of the principles and values that underpin both health-promotion theory and practice is also evident in this chapter. The discussion of health promotion is contextualised from an Irish perspective.

Chapter 2 deals specifically with the relationship between the development of public policy and health promotion. It examines planning in health-service provision and discusses the key contribution of a health-promotion ethos to public policy. The relationship between health promotion and public health is explored. It particularly concentrates on the influence of health promotion on the development of public policy from a national and international perspective. This chapter also critically analyses key national strategies that have influenced the development of health-promotion practice in Ireland.

Chapter 3 focuses on health promotion and change management. This chapter examines the theories that influence individual behavioural as well as community and organisational change. As change is a central element to most health-promotion work this chapter engages in an exploration of change theory, change processes and their relevance to health-promotion practice.

Chapter 4 examines empowerment as a core value in health-promotion theory and practice. The chapter offers a critical analysis of definitions of empowerment and discusses the role of power in the development of empowering relationships of practice. This chapter introduces the concepts of social capital and community development and their relationship to health promotion.

Chapter 5 explores health promotion, lifestyle issues and work. This chapter provides a framework within which to understand the relationship between lifestyle, behaviour and health. It debates the relationship between health and work and provides insights with regard to the dynamics of work–life balance. This chapter also examines the role of organisational culture in workplace health and looks at the role of workplace health-promotion initiatives.

Chapter 6 focuses specifically on current themes relevant to health-promotion practice. It provides an understanding of the contribution of sociology and psychology to health promotion and discusses the relationship between education and health promotion. The integration of health promotion into the practice of key professional groups is explored. It also explores health promotion with reference to multiculturalism and specific populations.

Section 2 provides the reader with the necessary basis to research, review and evaluate practice and programmes. This section begins with a discussion of evidence-based practice and the key paradigms underpinning research. It then introduces the reader to research approaches commensurate with health-promotion practice, such as phenomenology, critical theory, grounded theory and action research. The importance of evaluation in health promotion is explored. A discussion of ethics as central to good practice in research is included. In addition, this section provides practical guidance for health-promotion agents on research practice, conducting literature reviews, surveys, focus groups and interviews. A section providing practical tips on compiling a research proposal is also included.

The book offers students and practitioners a comprehensive exploration of health promotion. This text is of interest to students at undergraduate and postgraduate level. It is also aimed at health and social-service practitioners who engage in health promotion and health education. It is relevant to all those involved in the development of health management, social and public policy as well as students of and practitioners in the area of public health. It draws on exemplars from Irish and international situations to help the reader examine the practical significance of health-promotion theory with regard to work, community, public policy and organisational contexts.

Section 1
Health Promotion Theory and Principles

1

The Nature of Health and Health Promotion

Learning Outcomes:

On completion of this chapter the reader will be able to:

* understand the competing interests and influences on the definition of health
* discuss the domains of influence on health and health status
* debate the principles and values of health promotion
* discuss health promotion in an Irish context.

INTRODUCTION

This chapter explores definitions of health, illuminating the tensions inherent in current discourses regarding what constitutes health and wellbeing. It examines differing understandings of health approaches ranging from the medical approach to an empowerment one as influencing current developments in the health field. The domains of influence of health are discussed as they are particularly influential in health-promotion practice. Principles of health promotion are examined.

DEFINING HEALTH

Any consideration of health promotion should explore the concept of health before considering health promotion. While it might seem logical for there to be a single universally accepted understanding of health, this in fact is not the case. Likewise there is no unitary understanding of health promotion *per se*. We argue that in order to engage in health-promotion activities, it is necessary for practitioners to have a sound understanding of the theoretical underpinnings and focus of health promotion as a distinct area of interest.

It is important to understand that there are quite distinctive and divergent understandings of health. These understandings tend to reflect different approaches within healthcare disciplines as well as non-professional understandings. These definitional and conceptual differences have a long history. In fact, it can be argued that the differences in interpretation of the concept of health can be traced to early Grecian times, as epitomised in the contrasts between the Greek goddess Hygeia and the physician, Asclepius, who lived in the twelfth century BC.

Historical insights

Hygeia was a goddess who was worshiped because she was assumed to symbolise the virtues of wellbeing and wise lifestyles. Worshipers of Hygeia, in turn, believed that the role of the physician was to emphasise the benefits to be gained from following the laws of nature so as to ensure that mankind had both a healthy mind and a healthy body. In contrast Asclepius was a physician who epitomised a belief that the legitimate role of medicine was to treat disease (Tones and Green, 2004). In many ways this debate about the levels of interdependence and integration between mankind and the wider environmental conditions versus an emphasis on a disease-based understanding of health states has continued to be the issue of central divergence in defining health since that time.

The word health itself is a derivation of an Old English word, hael, meaning 'whole' (Naidoo and Wills, 2000). While the origins of the word clearly infer notions of 'wholeness'; 'completeness' and therefore comprehensiveness; in practice, the reality is that health has tended to be considered in dichotomous terms. It is either present or absent, or more specifically, reference is most likely to be made to either the presence or absence of disease. This trend also raises another important issue, namely who defines health? These are important issues to consider as a precursor to exploring health promotion.

Divergent conceptualisations of health

When, as a society, we require definitions, we tend to rely on 'expert' groups. Definitions of health offered by professional bodies or 'expert' groups clearly influence public or 'lay' understandings. Definitions and understandings of health vary between cultures and across time and are heavily influenced by such experts. Since the time of the French philosopher René Descartes in the seventeenth century, the influence of medicine as a discipline has been profound in terms of defining health-related conditions. This is hardly surprising, as medicine in Western societies in particular has held a dominant position in both health-related occupations and society since at least then. Medicine has long been accepted as a traditional profession whose knowledge of diseases is well respected.

Definitions of health and illness offered by medicine, in turn, are extremely influential both in terms of our understanding of health and deviations from health as well as how these conditions may best be treated or managed. Medicine has a legitimate and well-respected expertise with regard to the identification and treatment of illness, which represents a health deviation. However, it is arguable that medicine does not have exclusive, conceptual or operational expertise in matters of health. Indeed there is evidence that the field of health promotion has become a unifying approach drawing on professional and lay expertise – one that has remained separate from medicine, while drawing on its distinct knowledge.

There are several distinct ways of defining health and illness that reflect these conceptual differences. Lay definitions of health and illness commonly overlap with professional ones such as those offered by professional bodies and/or originating in esteemed bodies such as the World Health Organization (WHO). It is noteworthy that there are definitional differences between states of 'sickness' and 'disease' as well as 'illness' and 'wellbeing'. It is states of sickness, disease and arguably illness that are the predominant concerns of official health agencies both nationally and internationally. Therefore, it can be argued that it is somewhat incongruous that agencies which primarily deal with states of sickness, disease and illness are the very ones in whom society has vested responsibility for defining states of health and wellbeing.

While there is an increasing trend to reconceptualise health as a more holistic concept, there are a number of consistent themes running through many of the more traditional understandings of health. One of the common themes is that health is the 'absence of disease'. This is sometimes supported by the understanding that health is a 'complete state of wellbeing'. The issue here relates to the notion of 'completeness'. It is arguable that nobody ever achieves a complete state of wellbeing and that all states are comparative or relative.

Other definitions imply that health is a condition where adequate resources for living form the foundation of a healthy state.

Health as a state of being

Defining health as a 'state' is in itself problematic, as it suggests being in a particular 'state' at a static period in time and lacks dynamism. The divergence and diversity of emphasis in official definitions of health probably reflects the underlying philosophy or orientation of the agency offering the definition. Agencies and organisations that define health can be divided into those that understand health and illness from a biomedical perspective and those which have either a more holistic or at least social understanding of the concept.

In 1930 H. L. Mencken in the *American Mercury* (Mencken, 1949) proposed the following reflection on health. He asked:

> What is this thing called health? Simply a state in which the individual happens transiently to be perfectly adapted to his environment. Obviously, such states cannot be common, for the environment is in constant flux.

This proposition implies that there are a number of variables to be considered in any definition of health. Jones (1994) argues that health cannot be considered without recognition of the fact that it has physiological as well as psychological components, and at the same time is fundamentally a social state. In essence, Jones argues that while health and illness will, of course, be experienced by us at an individual level, our experiences of them are most likely to be understood by drawing on a stock of current social beliefs, ideas and practices.

A distinction needs to be drawn between states of health and illness and our reactions to these states. Sociological perspectives suggest that it is within the social institutions of contemporary society, such as the family and the education system, that we learn what health and illness are, as well as appropriate responses to them. In addition, the structures of power in society, such as the state welfare system, professional groups and social class, influence how we learn what it means to be 'sick', 'dependent' or 'disabled'. Our understandings of what it means to be either a 'patient' or a 'carer' are also influenced significantly by both the power structures and agencies of social control, such as medicine.

Mencken's (1949) reflection implies that health is essentially a state of being which occurs or develops at an individual level. In that sense, health can be understood as a state of being that is subject to wide individual variation as well as social and cultural interpretation. Health is also a state that is produced by the interplay of individual perceptions as well as social and environmental influences. Health should also be understood as dynamic in nature. While there are individual differences in terms of health, there are also likely to be temporal (across time) differences. Definitions of health by somebody at fifteen years of age are likely to be significantly different from those offered by somebody at sixty-five years of age. Differences in relation to the understanding of the concept of a health status have also been noted in relation to gender (Cox, 1985) as well as in relation to social role and occupational status (Jones, 1994).

Evolving definitions: the influence of the WHO

The World Health Organization has defined health in a number of ways since its inception. While these definitions have been dynamic and evolving, the changes have been more of emphasis than substance. In 1946 the World Health Organization defined health as 'a state of complete physical, mental and social well-being and not merely the absence of disease or infirmity' (WHO, 1946:2). Throughout the latter half of the twentieth century, health definitions have expanded to incorporate all aspects of living, including physical, mental, spiritual and social wellbeing.

This understanding provides an important expansion of the concepts of both health and wellbeing through the inclusion of areas such as spirituality. It seems on first inspection to equate the concept of health with wellbeing, and in addition broadens the concept from one which is primarily focused on physiological status to incorporate mental, spiritual and social aspects of life. This concept of health, which is almost a complete rejection of the notion of health as the absence of disease, has become a fairly standard approach to defining health used by health-service agencies. In addition it has been particularly influential in facilitating practitioners who wish to move the emphasis of their practice from an illness-treatment or management paradigm to one which places an emphasis on enhancement of health. However, as a definition, it poses virtually as many problems or challenges as it resolves.

This understanding of health can be seen as being somewhat idealistic, and even utopian. In effect this definition offers a state which is to be aspired to. While it introduces the notion of wellbeing, the suggestion is clearly that wellbeing is a state wherein there is balance and an integration of the four facets of health, and there is an inadequate exploration of the notion of wellbeing. The dynamic nature of definitions and concepts is obvious in the WHO's definition of health in 1984, in both the definition itself and in the rank order in which the various components of health are arranged.

This definition conceptualised health as:

> The extent to which an individual or group is able, on the one hand, to realise aspirations and safety needs and on the other hand, to change or cope with the environment. Health is therefore seen as a resource for everyday life, not the objective of living: it is a positive concept emphasising social and personal resources as well as physical capabilities.
>
> (World Health Organization 1984:23)

This definition of health is not as frequently quoted as the earlier one, but it contains developments and enhancements that need to be considered. In the first instance, health is not seen as an end in its own right. It is seen as a dynamic rather than a static entity, intrinsically linked with and underpinning everyday life. While it remains consistent with the earlier definition in rejecting the idea that health is merely the absence of disease, it also broadens the concept from an individual one to incorporate both individuals and groups. Interestingly it incorporates concepts of psychological and social functioning in that it clearly relates a state of health to coping mechanisms and strategies as well as the ability of individuals or groups to adapt within a particular environment. Health is also reconceptualised as a resource rather than an outcome. It confirms its dynamic as well as its multidimensional nature.

The World Health Organization in its *World Health Report* (WHO, 2001a) pointed out that since its inception it has always defined health as a multi-faceted phenomenon. This is undoubtedly true, though it is equally true that there has been refinement of the definition across time. Jones (1994) identifies a very interesting difficulty that this evolution in definition poses. Because the nature of health is multidimensional and a dynamic rather than a static concept, this means that it cannot be easily analysed and measured in an absolute way. Given the fact that healthcare professionals have traditionally understood health as an absence of disease and thus capable of measurement, this relatively recent change in emphasis challenges professional health workers' perspectives of health, which have stood for at least the past 150 years.

The efforts of bodies such as the World Health Organization to both define and refine definitions of health are quite important. As argued, many individuals rely on public and expert groups to define important concepts and then draw on those understandings themselves. However, not alone do individuals rely on expert-led definitions, governments and health-service agencies also do. One can see ongoing reference, for example, to WHO definitions in Government publications internationally. Governments and public-health bodies generally are the relevant agencies that drive public policy as well as implement it. Therefore inaccurate or inappropriate definitions can (at least potentially) lead to flawed policy and practice directions being followed, in relation to achieving greater health status among populations.

The understanding of the concept of health by policy makers influences the funding and operational direction of service providers. In that regard, understandings of both health and health promotion are important, for arriving at a shared understanding between official agencies, health professionals and individuals.

A more holistic or social model of health has emerged over the past half century that has influenced the public-health approach to healthcare services both nationally and internationally. Brennan (2000) argues that medicine began to take a firm control over the human processes of health from approximately the middle of the sixteenth century, with the publication of the first textbook of anatomy. Brennan also argues that professional medical organisations, which began to form in the nineteenth century, led the medical profession in their charge to control and develop a monopoly of health policy.

This monopoly can be seen to relate to health policy formation, implementation and evaluation. The model of health promoted by medicine is essentially a binary model, which locates health in a direct relationship with illness. This model held sway from at least the nineteenth century onwards and the evolving definitions offered by the World Health Organization challenge the conceptual underpinnings of health as understood by the binary medical model. For this reason alone they can be seen as very important developments. At first glance they would be seen to challenge the monolithic perspective of health implicit in a biomedical model and to be somewhat more holistic in nature. It could be argued that they emanate from modern thinking which values sociological, psychological and spiritual influences in a more equitable way. However, Brennan (2000) argues that in fact, these definitions simply return the understanding of health to ones which were in existence prior to the era when scientific positivism and its application to human experiences and processes held dominance.

FACTORS THAT INFLUENCE HEALTH

Up to this point, we have been concerned with conceptual aspects of health and the differing meanings attributed to health. The influences of professional groups on the evolution of consensus with regard to definitions of health have been pointed out as issues that need to be considered in deciding the merits of any definition. However, what is also evident is that health is a complex and multifaceted phenomenon that has meanings drawn from the biological or physical sciences, as well as sociological, psychological and related domains of knowledge. Given that this is the case, it is hardly surprising that there is a wide range of factors that influence health and health status. Many of these factors are referred to as 'determinants of health'. In itself, this term seems to imply that any or all of a range of factors impact on health status in a deterministic manner. This has tended to be an approach taken in health-related research in more recent times. It would however be somewhat naïve to assume that simplistic linear relationships on their own explain the complex interactions between individual characteristics and health-related manifestations.

While there are many more influences on health and health status, the primacy of individual responsibility for health remains popular. In many ways, this understanding of health and responsibility for health status reflects a divergence of opinion between those who subscribe to an ideology of individualism versus one of collectivism. However, the growing recognition of the importance of associated, multiple and/or interrelated factors influencing health is welcome for a number of reasons. Firstly, it acknowledges and understands health as both a complex and multifaceted phenomenon. Secondly it values the understanding and input of multiple disciplines and interest groups and thirdly, it is an approach that also makes sense.

This 'common sense' approach is welcome because it pragmatically recognises that there is a shared responsibility for health status as well as shared benefits between individuals and broader communities. Reflecting this more pragmatic understanding, Milio (1981) argued that lifestyle choices could not be independently made in a completely free manner and that the range of choices that constitute lifestyle patterns must be contextualised in the socioeconomic and environmental circumstances in which people find themselves. Consideration of a particular case might help to illustrate this.

JONATHAN'S STORY

Jonathan is a twelve-year-old boy who has recently been diagnosed with a complex metabolic disorder. In order that Jonathan can maintain a normal lifestyle, he requires routine dietary supplements and management of a cocktail of medication as well as regular visits to a specialist clinic. Jonathan's father is unemployed and both of his parents have limited literacy skills.

While the family are entitled to a medical card, neither parent knows how to apply for one. Likewise, they do not have a regular general practitioner. Claims for reimbursement for Jonathan's medication require regular contact with Health Board officials and forms to be filled.

Jonathan is unable to make the regular appointments at the specialist clinic in Dublin because he lives in an isolated location in a rural community with no regular public transport.

This story highlights the relationship and complex interaction between the individual, their environment and the resources available to them. It also points to the fact that 'being healthy' is something that can hardly be regarded as a static state. In addition, when we think about a 'state of health' we frequently also use as a point of comparison, a 'state of illness'. This is, however, not always a welcome thing as the concept of wellbeing is a factor that also needs to be considered and is implicit in the WHO definition.

Wellbeing refers to the person's ability to understand, accept, manage or cope with their own level of ability or functioning. It encompasses their worldview of their own situation, their perception of their health status in the context of their living arrangements and may be influenced by internal factors such as self-esteem, cognitive processes, knowledge and insight, among others. For example, someone who has a serious and enduring health deficit, such as insulin-dependent diabetes, may be considered objectively to be unhealthy. However, given the availability of insulin, the knowledge and skills to self-administer their medication, test, interpret and act on blood-sugar levels, understand the lifestyle factors as well as the sense of internal control of their own lives, most people in this situation have a very positive sense of wellbeing. In other words they can manage their own life situations and also have a sense of control over their own medical condition. In this context, we can begin to appreciate that health is complex, and that the factors that influence our health status are equally likely to be multifaceted.

Within medical science there has been a long tradition of enquiry into the factors that lead to illness. Epidemiology concerns itself with the factors that influence illness conditions. Indeed, a long-standing definition argues that epidemiology is 'the study of the distribution and determinants of disease in human populations' (Barker and Rose, 1984:5). It is equally understandable that health and social policy makers and society more generally should be concerned with similar factors that influence health and in turn have tended to rely on medicine for appropriate answers.

This argument has previously been made in the context of presenting an integrated approach to health-promotion activity and associated work in public-health nursing (McDonald, 2004). However, there are dangers in the inappropriate application of the principles of epidemiological investigation to health-promotion activities. Some of these dangers may be obvious in the trends within health promotion to concentrate on lifestyle and risk behaviours. These factors are also frequently referred to as 'health determinants', drawing on the traditions of epidemiological research associated with illness and disease.

Just as with any illness condition, the factors that influence health can probably be understood at both an individual and group level. In this section concentration will be placed on community- or societal-level influences.

Considering health determinants at a group level is consistent with a population-based approach to health. As with illness conditions, these approaches draw on epidemiological evidence, social and environmental trends and influences as well as individual factors. When examining health-related issues in any society, researchers have traditionally drawn on data such as morbidity and mortality statistics associated with particular conditions. For example, comparisons are commonly drawn between such factors as morbidity rates and heart conditions, lifestyle patterns and such variables as age or gender. This in itself is very beneficial in informing us about likely risk factors or the relationship between illness and service activity or usage. However, no matter how useful this information is in relation to the planning of services to provide for individuals with particular illnesses, it is extremely limited in terms of describing the influence of particular lifestyle choices on health as opposed to illness.

Within health-promotion literature a number of typologies or models of health determinants have been presented. For example, Simons-Morton, Green and Gottlieb (1995) argue that the determinants of health have tended to be divided into four broad categories, namely genetics, environment, healthcare and personal behaviour. These authors argue that this general framework is useful, but divide the environmental category into two, namely the physical and the social environment. Dahlgren and Whitehead (1991) had previously argued for a similar model suggesting that personal factors including age, sex and hereditary factors, as well as personal lifestyle factors, social networks and supports, living and working conditions and more global socioeconomic, cultural and environmental factors were the ones that influence health.

In considering a model of health determinants, individual factors are important. However, it is the transaction within and between these factors that forms the central component of understanding this model. This is also evident in the model suggested by Dahlgren and Whitehead (1991) when they refer to 'layers of influence on health'. There seems to be a great deal of commonality between these models, but it is questionable whether or not the use of terms such as 'determinant' is helpful. While there is little doubt that the use of such a term is consistent with the ethos of epidemiology, it is perhaps more correct to refer to the areas that impact on health status as 'domains of influence'. We believe that the factors that are most likely to impact on health status or the experience of health can be divided into the following domains:

- personal factors
- interpersonal factors
- micro-environmental factors
- broader sociopolitical/environmental factors

Figure 1.1 Domains of influence on health and health status

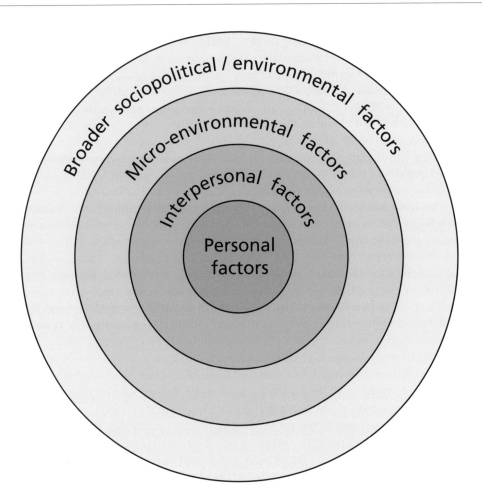

Personal factors

Personal factors might include one's genetic and biological endowment, age and gender. Genetic factors are clearly issues over which individuals have no control (in terms of predetermined influences). There are other personal factors over which individuals do have control to varying degrees. These would include cognitive processes (as opposed to ability); utilisation of physical capacity; locus of control, self-image, esteem and efficacy as examples.

Interpersonal factors

These factors can be described as those that include lifestyle, personal behaviour and interpersonal relationships within our immediate social milieu, as well as our health beliefs and expectations. Health beliefs and expectations can be completely personal, but are likely to be influenced by such factors as the level of information we have, peer influences and social experiences. These factors, therefore, are essentially interpersonal.

Micro-environmental factors

These refer to issues within our immediate environment, such as personal living conditions, employment status and conditions, standard of education achieved. Personal living conditions are influenced by issues such as income and wealth or poverty levels and are strongly related to health and illness status. While these will also most likely involve other people, they are distinguished from interpersonal factors in that interpersonal factors are largely associated with relationships with other people as opposed to our local environmental situation.

Broader sociopolitical environmental factors

These include the social and political environment in which individuals live, the educational standards within the society, the level and nature of health-service provision, governmental strategies and policies and social-service provision, and the social networks that influence people's lives. They also include national and international influences, trans-governmental factors, the economic influences on health and health status, as well as the political ethos, opportunities and choices available within society.

Clearly factors such as the political stability of a country are likely to influence health status as well as the social structures and opportunities available to individuals within particular cultures. The availability of essential services such as electricity, sanitation services, or indeed air and water quality as well as the built environment are all factors (both individually and in combination) that are likely to impact on individual and collective health status. Likewise, the availability of screening, preventative and curative health-related services will impact on health status. There is also fairly clear and long-standing evidence that social status or membership of particular social groupings is related to health status (Department of Health and Social Security, 1980; Combat Poverty Agency, 2003).

CURRENT TRENDS AND EMERGING CONSENSUS

Within an international as well as an Irish context, examination of the literature and national reports has tended to focus on lifestyle behaviours and the relationship between these factors and health or illness status. For example, in the Irish context, a Health Promotion Unit was established within the Department of Health and Children following the publication of the first national health-promotion strategy in Ireland in 1995 (*Making the Healthier Choice the Easier Choice*: DoHC, 1995). Following this, the Health Promotion Unit commissioned two studies, the Survey of Lifestyles, Attitudes and Nutrition (SLÁN) (Centre for Health Promotion Studies, 2003), focusing on adults, and Health Behaviour in School-aged Children (HBSC) (Centre for Health Promotion Studies, 1999).

These studies represented the first attempt in Ireland to gather focused data on health-related issues at a national level within a health-promotion context and were based on similar international approaches. The findings provided comprehensive baseline data. Interestingly, the domains that were focused upon in the SLÁN survey included 'attitudes towards or perceptions of general health, use of alcohol and other substances, food and nutrition, exercise and accidents' (Centre for Health Promotion Studies, 2003:4)

The concentration is clearly on lifestyle, with a focus on risk behaviours and the findings seem consistent with international trends. Focusing on individual lifestyle and risk behaviour is insufficient particularly as the domains of influence on health are much broader. There is emerging consensus that factors such as poverty, gender, ethnicity, social status and many others are related to health status. Indeed the importance of the interplay between individual behaviours and broader sociopolitical and environmental factors has been widely accepted since the Black Report (DHSS, 1980), which reported that there were health-related inequalities evident at every stage of life between traditional 'classes' or socioeconomic groupings.

For example, the Report found that those in the lower classes had higher death rates than those in the higher classes. It also reported that children born into lower social classes had lower birth rates and shorter stature, while all the major diseases affected social classes four and five more than one or two (the higher ones). It is reasonable to argue that the types of inequality evident between social 'classes' or based on demographic factors such as age, gender, class or ethnicity are ones that people interested in health promotion need to consider carefully. These factors should be seen as ones that reflect structural inequalities within broader society. This highlights the necessity to understand health promotion as an ethos as much as an activity.

In Ireland, similar inequities to those highlighted in the Black Report were reported by Nolan (1990) who found a disparity in mortality rates among those in the fifteen to sixty-four age group based on social class. Those described as 'higher professional' had a rate of mortality of thirteen per 1,000 population, while those described as 'semi-skilled manual' had a rate of twenty-two per 1,000, with those who were 'unskilled manual' having the highest mortality rate in this age category, with a death rate of thirty-two per 1,000 (Nolan, 1990).

TOWARDS A DEFINITION OF HEALTH PROMOTION

Health-promotion activities are certainly not new. Activities associated with promoting healthy lifestyles and reducing the risk or prevalence of illness and disease predate the notion and concept of 'health promotion'. Health Promotion as a distinct activity is in fact a phenomenon of the latter part of the twentieth century. Despite its conceptual longevity there is a lack of clarity about the actual term itself. Downie, Tannahill and Tannahill (1996) noted that:

> Health promotion is used in a number of different ways, even by the same people . . . It is perfectly possible – and indeed by no means uncommon – for two people, or even an entire committee or conference, to have a discussion about health promotion and be referring to very different things. In effect, health promotion has become a dazzling

bandwagon, gaining momentum, and with all and sundry clamoring to climb aboard, without giving sufficient thought to what it is and where it is going.

The phrase 'health promotion' comprises two words – health and promotion. The issue of health has already been explored. *The Concise Oxford Dictionary* proposes three meanings of the word 'promotion'. Firstly, promotion may be an activity that supports or encourages; secondly, it may be the publishing of a product or venture so as to increase sales or public awareness; thirdly, it may involve the action of raising somebody to higher position or rank or the fact of being so raised (Pearsall, 1999).

In the context of health promotion, all three components of this definition may be seen to apply. Within health promotion activity, both individuals and communities are supported and encouraged to select or engage in healthy lifestyle choices. Health promotion as an activity is published and publicised widely in order to both enhance public awareness and increase healthy lifestyles. The ultimate aim of health-promotion activity is, in fact, to raise individuals' and communities' health status. Therefore health promotion can be considered as the activity of supporting and encouraging the publishing and presentation of health-promoting activities as well as the raising of individuals and groups to a higher level of health status.

Another important issue which needs to be addressed is that of boundaries. Health, as we have seen, has a number of different aspects which need to be considered. These include individual behaviour, community participation and action as well as the environment. Based on the fact that health encompasses so many human activities, it is difficult at a conceptual level to place boundaries on health-promoting activities. The very fact of placing a boundary creates an artificial axis of activities that either are or are not health-promoting. However, if boundaries are not identified then all activity associated with living can be associated with health promotion. Adopting this model can create a situation where a range of activities may be expressed as health-promotion activities for political expediency, but in reality may not be health-promoting. In addition a term loosely defined in this way which has such a potentially diffuse or diverse meaning can be used to refer to everything, and in turn ends up meaning nothing.

The politicisation of health-promotion activities is obvious from the period of the 1980s onwards. Throughout this period, a range of new jargon emerged in the health-related field. The concepts of health promotion, patient advocacy and community care all emerged as new concepts. However, we would argue that in fact they were not new concepts but in many cases were revised, modified or changed terms for carrying out the same activity in a different setting. In relation to what emerged as health promotion, much of the activity remained the same but was labelled as health promotion. Prior to this time, much health-promotion activity was simply information-giving. Information-giving as an activity was already in existence but was subsumed into the term health promotion. This activity relied on the same approaches that had been used previously and was based on the same assumptions about people's lifestyles as when it was called 'health education'.

Health education is one facet of health-promotion activity. If an activity is to be defined as health-promoting, there must be at least some degree of the purposeful pursuit of a realisable health gain. This distinction is important in helping to clearly define the nature of health-promotion processes. While the boundaries of what constitutes health promotion should be clearly defined, it is equally important to establish the scope of health promotion. In this regard, the areas of life in which health promotion can occur are both varied and interlinked.

Integration is central to the health-promotion approach. Health promotion can be viewed as a set of integrated activities which are responsive to the perceptions, needs and desires of individuals and communities (Brennan, 2000). Activities which are not integrated and which do not have community participation may therefore be considered as ones which, while worthwhile in their own right, are outside the boundaries of the concept of health promotion. Therefore both the scope and boundaries of health promotion may be encapsulated in the belief that health promotion comprises a purposeful health-oriented action that is integrated in nature and takes cognisance of and encourages community participation. Thus, health promotion may occur at an individual, community, national, international or indeed planetary level. From a policy perspective, a wide variety of government departments as well as voluntary agencies and local bodies have a legitimate concern, interest and contribution to health-promotion activities.

Internationally, the focus on illness prevention predates the notion of formal health-promotion activity, though there is clearly a degree of overlap and shared interest between them. For example, in the United States, the Surgeon General published a report in 1980 titled *Healthy People: The Surgeon General's Report on Health Promotion and Disease Prevention* (Department of Health and Human Services, 1980a). Clearly the conceptual link between the promotion of health as a means of preventing illness is evident in the title of this report. This trend was also evident in other reports produced in the US up to 1990, for example, *Promoting Health/Preventing Disease: Objectives for the Nation* (1980b) followed by *Healthy People 2000: National Health Promotion and Disease Prevention Objectives* (1990).

The agenda for health-promotion activities within a European context has largely been outlined and determined by the World Health Organization in recent times. The WHO endeavoured to realise its aspiration of 'Health for all by the year 2000' (WHO, 1978). This particular policy set out targets and strategies which were underpinned by the principles of equity, empowerment and participation with a focus on the delivery of care in a primary-care setting and based on multidisciplinary and inter-agency working models.

Health promotion as a structured approach can be generally dated to a series of declarations and conferences from 1978 onwards. In 1978, the International Conference on Primary Care resulted in the Declaration of Alma Ata, which is generally credited as being the formal international initiation point in terms of the setting of health-related goals and international commitments to the attainment of its goal of 'Health for all by the year 2000'. This Declaration comprised ten sections and while generally credited with focusing on 'primary healthcare', it is interesting that many of the statements contained in the Declaration have a very firm 'health promotion' ethos. For example the Declaration asserts the highest possible level of health as a fundamental human right; it refers to health inequalities as being related to economic, social and political issues and argues that the promotion and protection of health is essential for economic and social development, quality of life and even world peace. It advocated that primary healthcare was the medium through which acceptable global health status would be achieved by 2000 and into the period beyond.

This Declaration was built on in 1986 when the first International Conference on Health Promotion in Ottawa presented a charter of action points to meet the objectives of achieving 'Health for all by the year 2000 and beyond' (WHO, 1986). This charter refined the definition of health. While it reaffirmed health as being a *state* of complete physical, mental and social wellbeing, it also referred to health as being a *resource* for everyday life rather than an objective in its own right. It argued that a state of health was a positive concept that emphasised social as well as personal resources in addition to physical capacities. This clearly stressed a broad, holistic and social model of health and in that regard recognised that attainment of health was not the sole prerogative of the 'health sector'. The Ottawa Charter identified eight fundamental prerequisites for health, namely: peace, shelter, education, food, income, a stable eco-system, sustainable resources as well as social justice and equity. These factors are not the sole preserve or responsibility of the traditional health sector.

Based on this conceptualisation of health, the Charter defined health promotion as:

the process of enabling people to increase control over, and to improve, their health. To reach a state of complete physical, mental and social well-being, an individual or group must be able to identify and to realize aspirations, to satisfy needs, and to change or cope with the environment. Health is, therefore, seen as a resource for everyday life, not the objective of living. Health is a positive concept emphasizing social and personal resources, as well as physical capacities. Therefore, health promotion goes beyond healthy life-styles to well-being.

(WHO, 1986)

This definition emphasises the significance of healthy lifestyles but is not limited to lifestyle or behaviour issues only. The Charter advocates that health-promotion action incorporates the building of healthy public policy, the creation of supportive environments, strengthening community actions, developing personal skills and the reorientation of health services (WHO, 1986). This Charter has been the predominant influence on health-promotion activity in the intervening period.

PRINCIPLES AND APPROACHES TO HEALTH PROMOTION

A range of approaches to health promotion is evident in the literature, with some key distinctions evident between them. These approaches are influenced by a number of factors. For example the professional background of practitioners influences practice, as does the political, social and economic climate and the ethos of the country or location in which health promotion is practised (or not). Health-promotion activity and initiatives will include programmes, policies and other organised activities that adhere to a number of key principles. These include empowerment, participation, holism, intersectoral collaboration, and should be multi-strategy in nature. Health-promotion approaches are also characterised by their commitment to advocacy, equity and sustainability.

The approaches to health promotion have been hugely influenced by the fact that medicine has been the dominant model within health-service provision and a clear division exists between those who support the medical model of health and those who argue for a more holistic and/or social model of health. Therefore, the importance of understanding the influence of differing models should be obvious.

Models (in the simplest understanding of the term), just like model cars or railways or building models, provide us with a means of understanding or conceptualising a complex and larger entity. They help us to comprehend reality or to integrate complex issues into a representation that is more understandable. Within health services, models of care are fairly well understood and well established as conceptual entities. For example, within nursing, a wide range of formal models of nursing have been developed for well over the past half-century. These models are assumed to provide an explanation of the relationship between different facets of nursing, for example, understandings of nursing, health, 'personhood', the environment and the interrelationship between these domains of practice (Pearson *et al.*, 1996). The evolution of these models is largely assumed to help nursing base its practice on unique theories and advance the professionalisation of nursing.

In a similar way, a range of theories and conceptual understanding of health promotion has evolved and for similar reasons. Both the theories and models that underpin health promotion as an activity or an ethos are essentially focused at individual, interpersonal and community levels. Within these domains there are a number of prominent key models. The models and theories reflect either an individual focus or explanation of health promotion or alternatively interpersonal or community approaches.

EMPOWERMENT AS A UNIFYING THEME IN HEALTH PROMOTION

Empowerment is central to health promotion and has been a core principle upon which health-promotion activity has been based since the Ottawa Charter. It has assumed greater importance in subsequent global conferences on health promotion. At the fifth global conference held in Mexico City in 2000, the imperative of empowerment was evident in the title of the conference itself: 'Health Promotion; Bridging the Equity Gap'. The concept of equity, or more precisely inequity (where a 'gap' needs to be bridged) is essential to the empowerment process.

Power and equity are concepts that are both closely related to the fields of sociology and social psychology. Power, the exercise of power and power imbalance are generally seen as resting within the domains of the individual, the community and the state. Increasing levels of influence and power are evident from international sources. When power is understood to incorporate influence, or manifests itself as such, the macro-level extends not only to international bodies and agencies, but increasingly to sources of information such as the internet and the actions and lifestyles portrayed by international stars, including those of screen, stage, sport and politics. The work of health promotion is mandated to some extent by both the Jakarta (WHO, 1997) and Mexico Declarations (WHO, 2000) to incorporate into its work social responsibility for health. This, in essence, provides the basis for sociopolitical work and the types of social, political as well as individual advocacy that underpin the empowerment approach to health promotion.

Tones and Green (2004) argue rather convincingly that an empowerment model of health promotion underpins all domains of health. An empowerment approach to health promotion is one that is congruent with all the principles of health promotion, as outlined earlier. Their work argues that the central dynamic of such a model relates to the interplay between the traditions of health education and healthy public policy.

This theme is also taken up by Whitehead (2004) who argues that the traditional differences between health education and promotion lie more in emphasis and methods than anything else. In fact, the traditions of health education and information-giving were based on principles of empowerment. In that case the empowerment was understood to be obtained through the provision of information, which would 'empower' the individual to make 'healthy choices'. The main weakness inherent in that approach is that individuals were both the focus of attention and indeed the medium for change. With increasing recognition of the importance of other players (or as we refer to them, domains of influence) the relevance of empowerment approaches to populations, settings, agencies, governments and inter-governmental agencies becomes obvious as does the limitation of focusing exclusively on individuals for change.

The empowerment approach suggests two main strategies for health promotion; firstly through traditional advocacy or mediation approaches and secondly through political agitation and action (Tones and Green, 2004). In the context of an empowerment approach, however, these authors very clearly argue that the type of mediation and advocacy undertaken should be within the understanding that the actions taken by health-promotion agents fit within a particular framework. They argue that health promoters are in a powerful position and that as persons with power, their lobbying of those who exercise power is undertaken on behalf of those with limited power (or none).

This distinction is important and requires careful consideration and ongoing monitoring. There is always the possibility that boundaries of self versus selfless interest may be transgressed. From a sociological perspective, there is a danger that health-promotion agents will emerge as an elite themselves and as a 'professional group' or discipline, there are likely to be professional interests and agendas that will also need to be promoted. In that regard, a key factor that requires constant vigilance relates to the question of when, for example, are health-promotion agents acting solely on behalf of others and when are there possibilities that as a 'professional group' the interests of the group coincide with or supersede the interests of the group being represented?

ADVOCACY IN HEALTH PROMOTION

Tones and Green (2004:38) provide a useful conceptualisation of advocacy, as the 'Lobbying of those who exercise power by those who have power but who are doing so on behalf of the relatively powerless'. Advocacy has gained increasing currency in health-related services and debates and this development is generally seen as welcome and positive. In many ways it can be argued that advocacy has its origins in the consumer movement and that it provides 'a voice' for vulnerable or less powerful individuals and groups. Within the context of the definition given by Tones and Green (2004), advocacy is seen as being undertaken by a powerful group or individual on behalf of less powerful individuals or groups. In itself, while this can be presented as an admirable activity, it assumes that no other agendas are being pursued by the advocate(s) and it presumes altruism underpins the activity.

However, it does not seem reasonable to assume that the interests of professional or other interest groups can be completely ignored, or indeed altruism assumed as the sole guiding factor in advocacy roles. Since its inception as an approach within health promotion, many interests and professional groups have effectively been in competition, each claiming advocacy as a key area of interest, activity or influence. This means that competing interests may also be involved in 'turf claiming' and may cloud the capacity for altruistic advocacy. Examination of the professional groups who claim to have an interest in health promotion may help illustrate this point. In the late 1980s it was argued that those with an interest in, or more importantly claiming ownership of, the concept of health promotion included health and education professionals, behavioural and social scientists, holistic health and self-care advocates, liberals, conservatives, voluntary associations, funding agencies, governments, community groups and others (Green and Raeburn, 1988:30). The diversity of interests, agendas or perspectives among these groups should be self evident, when examined in the context of the definition of advocacy by Tones and Green (2004). Despite the possible contradictions and competing interests within or between these groups, there is a general consensus that advocacy is an important element of health-promotion activity as well as an ethos.

HEALTH PROMOTION IN THE IRISH CONTEXT

When considering health promotion in an Irish context, it is important to remind ourselves that health promotion in a formal sense is a relatively recent phenomenon. As indicated earlier, the international emphasis on health promotion as an approach dates from the 1980s in most instances.

The first formal governmental strategy on health promotion was published in Ireland in 1995 (DoHC, 1995). This document followed the publication of the first national strategy on health ever published: *Shaping a Healthier Future* (DoHC, 1994). *Shaping a Healthier Future* both provided the context for health-service development for a defined period and introduced language that indicated at least a governmental desire to base health services on a more social model of health. It also demonstrated some evidence of a health-promoting ethos. However the existing trends towards health promotion prior to 1995 also need to be acknowledged.

The national health strategy (DoHC, 1994) set out specific principles and argued for the necessity for a reorientation of health services. The first national health promotion strategy (DoHC, 1995) adopted a similar approach. It identified specific targets and placed a strong value on measurable outcomes. This must be understood in the context of ongoing political and public concerns about the perceived failure of health services to deliver quality services, while simultaneously using increasing proportions of public funding. The national health strategy (1994), in turn, emphasised accountability, a reorientation of the health services, an emphasis on consumer involvement and greater levels of access and equity. This strategy also introduced the term 'health and social gain' into the lexicon of Irish public policy.

The 1995 health promotion strategy, as indicated, also adopted a target-focused approach. It clearly identified the specific areas where health-promotion activity would be undertaken, for example, communities, schools and work settings as well as the health services themselves. This, from a historical perspective, was important in that it formally recognised that the settings related to health were more diverse than just the health-service setting traditionally associated with health in Ireland. This shift of policy direction was diametrically opposed to the trends of some twenty-odd years and the very conceptual basis on which the health services were organised under the Health Act (1970). In the white paper that preceded that Act, the rationale provided for the regionalisation of services was (at least partly) to facilitate centralisation and rationalisation of services as well as the development of centres of excellence in terms of 'medical' care. This was consistent with the principles of providing an 'expert'-driven service, rather than a consumer-driven one. Given that the very basis of the organisational structure of services was being formally challenged, this document provides an important reference point to health promotion in Ireland.

A second *National Health Promotion Strategy* was published in 2000 (DoHC, 2000) and this strategy can be seen as a progression of the 1995 document in a number of ways. In the second strategy the requirement for intersectoral collaboration was expanded upon, with much stronger emphasis placed on the role of factors outside the direct control or remit of traditional health services in influencing health. In addition, the dominance of the medical influence on health services was challenged in that a multidisciplinary approach was also promoted, while the limitations of a purely biomedical understanding of, or approach to, health were clearly evident. The strategy was to be implemented between 2000 and 2005. In a review of the strategy (DoHC, 2004c), significant progress in its implementation was noted.

Up to relatively recent times, health promotion in Ireland has been seen as a somewhat discrete 'activity'. However, this understanding is somewhat limited, and arguably reductionist in nature. Health promotion, of course, involves specific activities, but it is essentially an ethos and approach to health which has implications for health-service organisation and delivery.

While health promotion is an approach rather than a specific activity, one of the means of auditing governmental commitment to health promotion is evident in the allocation of resources to health promotion as opposed to illness prevention or illness-management services. It must be acknowledged, however, that informal health-promotion activity should be integral to all forms of illness prevention and treatment approaches.

In that regard, the Department of Health and Children (2004) identified a total of 307 staff employed in the public health system nationally. Of those, 142 were in jobs with the titles Health Promotion Officer, Senior Health Promotion Officer or Health Promotion Manager. The rest included dieticians (forty-six), drug services (twenty-nine) and other positions (ninety). These positions include a range of administrative grades as well as smoking-cessation facilitators etc.

Examination of the work of many of those included within the overall total would reveal that much of the practice of those involved in drug services and 'other positions' is focused on rehabilitation and intervention services as much if not more than health-promotion activity. Therefore, it can be argued that this may over-represent the true situation in relation to dedicated health-promotion posts.

Besides formal health-promotion strategies, it is also worth noting that there is evidence of health-promotion principles in other health-policy and related activity in an Irish context. As mentioned, since 1994 Ireland's health policy has been guided by two national health strategies. Both of these documents actively promote a multisectoral approach to health-service provision and acknowledge the relationship between health, social and environmental factors as well as the role of broader governmental actions or indeed inactions.

In relation to the more recent strategy *Quality and Fairness: A Health System for You* (DoHC, 2001b), the specific aims for the health services are interesting. It argues that we should have a health system that:
- supports and empowers individuals, families and communities in achieving their full health potential
- is there when it is needed, is fair and is trustworthy
- encourages consumers to have their say, is responsive and ensures that consumers' views are taken into account.

Additionally, it is based on four principles, namely: equity, people-centredness, quality of care and clear accountability. All these guiding principles were also in the 1994 strategy, with people-centredness being the only one added in 2001. This suggests continuity and development simultaneously. *Quality and Fairness* also focuses to a greater extent on the domains of influence and argues for intersectoral approaches and the creation of supportive environments and a population focus for vulnerable groups in addressing health inequalities. The document identifies specific goals and highlights areas where change is required. The four national goals that are identified are:
- better health for everyone
- fair access
- responsive and appropriate care delivery
- high performance.

While these goals predominantly concentrate on health-service issues, the first goal is in fact for better health for the whole population. This pre-eminent goal has, of course, clear implications for health-promotional activities and intersectoral co-ordination is identified as the means through which this will be achieved.

Within the context of the health services, the strategy identifies a number of areas for reform. These include:

- strengthening primary care
- reform of the acute hospital system
- funding the health services
- developing human resources
- organisational reform
- developing health information.

Again, while many of the areas prioritised for reform and action relate to direct health-service provision, what is clear is that the reform is directed at refocusing the health services from expert-driven hospital-based intervention services, to a service that is more person- and client-centred. Specifically these reforms were intended to address issues of equity in eligibility for services, access to services as well as increased responsiveness and appropriateness of care. These reforms above all were also directed at improving system performance from a consumer perspective.

It is worth recalling that the World Health Organization has identified the principles of health promotion as including:

- empowerment of the whole population to take control of and be responsible for their own health
- tackling the determinants of health, including issues such as environment, poverty and social isolation
- intersectoral approaches to health involving a diverse range of sectors and governmental agencies and including legislation, economic and fiscal responses, organisational change, community development and educational approaches
- capacity-building at individual and community levels
- development of advocacy and educational roles for health professionals (WHO, 1984).

The Ottawa Charter for Health Promotion outlined five areas for action which provide a framework for all health-promotion activities:

- building healthy public policy
- creation of supportive environments
- strengthening of community action
- development of personal skills
- reorientation of the health services (WHO, 1986).

The national strategy currently in place seems to be embedded in these principles and approaches. However, not all actions of government and health services are consistent with an integrated approach or indeed with the principles of community empowerment. Despite over a decade of policy and strategy documents acknowledging the primacy of health promotion, and the value of taking cognisance of the determinants of health as the central focus of policy, it is somewhat disappointing that the fourth report of the Chief Medical Officer concentrates on lifestyle issues, based on an argument that lifestyle issues such as alcohol consumption, smoking and nutrition have a serious impact on public health and simultaneously that 'prevention is the cornerstone of any rational health policy' (DoHC, 2004a:5).

Despite the fact that there are legitimate concerns about health-service utilisation and lifestyle behaviours, this report, titled *Better Health through Prevention*, could be seen as inferring a conceptual link between lifestyle behaviour, public health, health-service provision and preventative measures and does not seem in keeping with more modern approaches to health promotion. While the report emphasises prevention and the introduction argues for health through prevention, many of the actions presented by the Chief Medical Officer actually focus on specific lifestyle topics and (as in the case of alcohol consumption) argue for intersectoral responses that are more in keeping with health-promotional activities than prevention *per se*. Other key strategies have also been published at national level. Perhaps the most influential of these from a health-promotion perspective has been the cardiovascular strategy (DoHC, 1999). This strategy has been very influential in workplace health-promotion initiatives.

The trend towards a health-promotion ethos of intersectoral collaboration is also obvious in other areas. Perhaps the medium through which the impact of healthy public policy has been most evident has been through this series of national agreements. In their original incarnation, these agreements concentrated almost exclusively on issues of pay and working conditions and were referred to as national wage agreements in the 1970s. These agreements subsequently evolved into a series of national understandings and, following a break between 1981 and 1987, a series of successive three-year national agreements emerged and formed a central tenet of public policy between government and the key social partners. The original partners were primarily the trade unions, employers and government. However, in more recent agreements the stakeholders have expanded to include representatives of the farming community as well as those in the voluntary and social sector.

This social partnership model is increasingly credited as a major contributory element to the success of the Irish economy in recent years. In the broader social arena, the *National Action Plan against Poverty and Social Exclusion 2003–2005* has as its key aim 'to build a fair and inclusive society and ensure that people have the resources and opportunities to live life with dignity and have access to the quality public services that underpin life chances and experiences' (Office for Social Inclusion, 2003:22). This clearly reflects a health-promotion influence and ethos.

The most recent agreement, *Sustaining Progress 2003–2005* (Government of Ireland, 2003) also incorporates ten key areas for special initiatives. These include housing and accommodation; the cost and availability of insurance; migration and interculturalism; long-term unemployment; vulnerable workers and those who have been made redundant; educational disadvantage; waste management; care issues with children, persons with disabilities and older people; alcohol and drug misuse; including everyone in the information society and ending child poverty. While it can be argued that these issues impact on the economy, they are consistent with principles of healthy public policy.

The mid-term review of *Sustaining Progress 2003–2005* refers to the concept of 'a successful society'. This implies a much broader understanding of social functioning and inclusiveness than would have been the case in relation to its precursors. The report argues that a successful society is underpinned by a dynamic economy, a participatory society, a commitment to social justice, consistent economic development that is socially and environmentally sustainable and responsiveness to the constantly evolving requirements of international competitiveness (Department of the Taoiseach, 2004).

The concept of 'healthy public policies' and concern for them is largely based on the assumption that the broader environmental context (including the social milieu) is one of the key domains of influence on health and social status. Therefore concern with, as well as the development of, 'healthy public policies' is an important component of health promotion, and is evidence of the impact of the health-promotion ethos permeating public policy. Governmental concern with such issues as environmental controls, agricultural standards, food production as well as processing and distribution, pollution, public transport, carbon emissions and housing policies among others, are ones that impact on the health and social status of individuals, groups and ultimately society. Recognition of the interrelatedness of economic and social interests is also consistent with the principles of healthy public policy. These ways of understanding health as an important contributory factor to social and economic functioning are at considerable variance with more traditional reductionist approaches. The fact that these principles are evident in a wide range of policies suggests that *healthy* public policy has been successfully incorporated, at least notionally, into Irish public policy.

2
Health Promotion and Public Policy

Learning Outcomes:

On completion of this chapter the reader will be able to:
- understand the concept of planning in health-service provision
- discuss the key contribution of a health-promotion ethos to public policy
- debate the impact of health promotion on public health from a national and international perspective
- critically discuss the key national strategies in the context of health promotion.

INTRODUCTION

Chapter 1 establishes the multifaceted nature of health and the complex interplay between individuals and the broader context in which they live. Chapter 1 also establishes that health promotion has evolved into a broadly sociopolitical endeavour which differs from the ethos and activity of traditional medically dominated health practice. Therefore, it is important to examine the factors that contribute to and influence social and public policy. This chapter will focus on strategic planning and strategies for health and social gain. It will examine the link between national and international policy and strategic developments and the impact they have on effective health promotion practice.

DEFINING PLANNING AND STRATEGIC INITIATIVES

Planning is an essential function of management. Not alone is it a right of managers to plan, it is an obligation that they do so. Planning and influencing policy and strategic development are at the very core of the ethos of health promotion. The principles of health promotion can only be realistically achieved through the adoption of a strategic approach to planning and policy development. It is through such means that health-promotion agents or professionals can achieve their goals.

One of the major criticisms of health-service planning has been that it has tended to be *ad hoc*, reactionary, unco-ordinated, expert-driven and thus disempowering in nature. Health-service development and delivery has not been short of plans, reviews and reports. It is arguable, however, that these plans lacked coherence and were expert-driven rather than consumer-led, which runs counter to the principles of social models of both health and health promotion.

It is also worth reiterating that the Ottawa Charter, which outlines the key areas for action for all health-promotion activities, mandates health-promotion professionals and activity to have a central role in planning and development. In fact only one of the five areas (listed below) for action can be seen as not directly related to planning and policy matters, that is, the development of personal skills:

- building healthy public policy
- creation of supportive environments
- strengthening of community action
- development of personal skills
- reorientation of the health services (WHO, 1986).

One of the areas of greatest contention in health services has been the development of somewhat polarised ideologies, which impact on the health of individuals and societies. This division can be characterised as one that distinguishes between individualism and collectivism. In the context of health, individualism essentially proposes individual responsibility for health and wellbeing as well as the conditions that underpin health. It presupposes that individual lifestyles and attitudes are the fundamental determinants of health and illness. Likewise, individuals have both the right as well as the freedom and responsibility to change their lifestyle to achieve an improved health status.

Individualism rejects the contention that health or illness are social products. It assumes that people have a free and indeed an informed choice, a stance that has been heavily criticised. Supporters of individualism tend not to question broader reasons or influences on issues such as risky behaviours (such as smoking or drinking to excess or having multiple sexual partners). They base their ideology on the assumption of both personal choice and the related assumption that choice can be reversed towards a healthier way of living.

Conversely, collectivism is based on the underlying belief that in many cases individuals do not have the power to change their lifestyles or their circumstances and that they can be empowered through a healthy public policy approach. Indeed, Milio (1981) suggests that patterns of personal behaviour cannot be understood outside of their context and are not a consequence of complete free choice. Milio argues that personal behaviours reflect choices selected from a range of alternatives. Choices are made on a complex basis and result from consideration of the socioeconomic situations people find themselves in and the ease with which they can make their choices (Milio, 1981).

Both perspectives can be criticised for their understanding of behaviour, approach and influence. For example, it can be argued that the ideology of individualism can result in victimisation and blaming. Individuals do not operate in a vacuum or a context-free environment. Equally, collectivism can be criticised for not holding individuals accountable for their own actions and being based on a (perhaps flawed) assumption that that people are invariably altruistic. In that regard, it has been criticised for its utopian principles (Beattie, 1991).

In many ways it is the imperative of health promotion to bridge this divide and consider individual functioning within the context of broader sociological or environmental perspectives. This trend is evident in the following refinements of the definition of the scope of health promotion. The original mandate from Ottawa argued that:

> advocacy for health, holism, enabling people to achieve their fullest potential and mediation of differing societal interests are cornerstones of health promotion.
>
> (WHO, 1986)

This was followed by the catchy phrase, which has persisted across time, arguing that health promotion was essentially concerned with 'making the healthier choice the easier choice' (Milio, 1986).

A rather interesting definition of the scope of health promotion was subsequently suggested by Tones, who incorporated the notion of 'handling disease' as well as all measures designed to promote health.

> Health promotion incorporates all measures deliberately designed to promote health and handle disease . . . a major feature of health promotion is undoubtedly the importance of 'healthy public policy' with its potential for achieving social change via legislation, fiscal, economic and other forms of 'environmental engineering'.
>
> (Tones, 1990)

This all-inclusive ethos is also contained in the definition by Tones and Green (2004). Interestingly in this definition the notions of holism and an 'upstream approach to prevention' are also incorporated:

> health promotion is a comprehensive approach that includes working at all levels and across all sectors. It involves a holistic view of health and well-being, a socio-ecological analysis of the determinants of health and an upstream approach to prevention.
>
> (Tones and Green, 2004:341)

Despite variation in emphasis across time, policy and planning involvement are consistent and central features of definitions of the scope and role of health promotion.

SOCIAL AND PUBLIC POLICY

The issue of public policy must form a central element of the discourse relating to the legitimate role of health promotion in policy formulation and implementation. Public policy, and in particular 'healthy' public policy is a central element of health promotion. Health promotion adopts as a central tenet the importance of social and environmental influences on health as much, if not more, than individual factors (Tones and Green, 2004). The importance of public policy cannot be understated. The term public policy is frequently used interchangeably with 'social policy'. Social policy was defined by the National Economic and Social Council (NESC) as:

> Those actions of government which deliberately or accidentally affect the distribution of resources, status, opportunities and life chances among social groups and categories of people within the country and thus help to shape the general character and equity of its social relations.
>
> (NESC, 1983:32)

This definition would seem to suggest that virtually all government policies or programmes have some implications for the wellbeing of the population. However, it has also been recommended that the term 'social policy' should be restricted to five broad areas comprising income maintenance, housing, education, health and welfare services (Curry, 1998).

This seems consistent with the subsequent assertion of the NESC (1981) in relation to the role of government through social policy initiatives. It then argued that traditionally, government actions, by means of social policy, occurred in response to four factors, namely the distribution of income, the provision of certain goods and services, states of dependency and notions of citizenship.

Social policy and the provision of social services can be seen as being part of a broader expression of social cohesion and solidarity. They also reflect the aspirations and norms of a given society. In the Irish context as well as the broader European one, there is evidence of increased levels of state intervention and broader use of public policy to impact on social and environmental conditions. This is perhaps particularly evident in the areas of health and social services. In the mid-1970s the principle aims of governmental interventions in social policy were directed to the relief of poverty and the provision of a minimum standard of living for all, the equalisation of opportunity and increased productivity and economic growth (Government of Ireland, 1970).

This in itself is an interesting commentary on the traditional focus of government action, which predates most formal 'health promotion' activity. The links between relief of poverty with opportunity and social status, productivity and economic performance is noteworthy. Within an Irish context, this linkage subsequently formed the basis of a range of social partnership arrangements that originally concentrated on pay and working conditions. These national agreements between the key social partners have frequently been cited as major contributors to the economic development and performance of the late twentieth and early twenty-first centuries.

These agreements expanded to incorporate issues of social inclusion and cohesion as well as matters relating to pay and working conditions. Therefore it can be argued that there has been a fairly dramatic increase in terms of intervention from a strategic and public-policy perspective in recent years. When we consider health and social issues, there has been a much longer tradition of intervention.

From at least the middle of the nineteenth century, the state has taken on an increasing responsibility for the direct and indirect provision of health services and their funding. One of the easiest, albeit simplistic, ways to gauge increases or decreases in intervention by government is to consider issues of expenditure. In that regard Wiley (1998) noted some interesting trends. For example, from the late 1940s onwards, the expenditure on health in Ireland increased by over thirty per cent of GNP in each decade until the 1980s (Wiley, 1997). The situation at the end of the twentieth century contrasted sharply with the early 1900s. From a health (or more precisely an illness) perspective, governmental involvement in 1900 was largely limited to preventing or controlling the spread or outbreak of the most serious contagious or epidemic diseases as well as ensuring access by the poor or destitute to general practitioner services, mainly through the dispensary system (Barrington, 1987).

Up to the formation of the Free State and indeed beyond, the health system had largely been a locally controlled and funded system. However this changed in an incremental manner to an increasingly centralised structure that is largely centrally financed. State health services in Ireland were first provided in a somewhat rudimentary manner under the Poor Law (Ireland) Act 1838. This legislation provided for infirmaries and other forms of medical care in association with the workhouses established in each Poor Law Union. Poor Law Unions were administrative units and there was a total of 126 unions in the Irish Republic. In 1851 the Unions were further divided into dispensary districts. Each Union had a physician attached to it who had responsibility to attend, without charge, to the sick and poor in the area. The dispensary system survived up to 1972.

In 1872 the Irish Local Government Board replaced the Irish Poor Law Commissioners. This system assumed control of both Poor Law and health services. In 1924, following the establishment of the Irish Free State, a government department titled the Department of Local Government and Public Health was established. The department continued as a unitary entity until 1947, when it was divided into the three distinct departments of local government, health and social welfare.

By 1947, therefore, a full government department had assumed responsibility for health, although again the focus of the work of that department was primarily on medical services. In 1970 a new Health Act was enacted which brought about regionalisation of health functions. Through this Act, eight health boards were established nationally, namely the Eastern, Western, Southern, Mid-Western, North-Eastern, North-Western, Midland and South-Eastern Health Boards.

From a public policy perspective, the rationale presented for this move to centralisation is interesting. In the white paper (1966), it is pointed out that the state had taken over the major share of the costs of running the services which were increasing substantially every year. It was therefore desirable to have a new administrative framework to combine national and local interest. This linkage between costs and administration suggests an economic imperative in health-service administration, but equally a concern was expressed that there was a need to match national need with local demand. This apparent conflict between local demand and national need seems contradictory to health-promotion principles of community involvement and empowerment.

Another reason cited in that white paper was that it was becoming more and more obvious that in order to develop the *medical service* itself, especially in relation to acute hospital care, it would be necessary to have the organisation on an inter-county basis. It was argued that the county as a unit was unsuitable as single counties were too small as an area for hospital services. Again the suggestion of the economic reality taking precedence over the involvement of a local community was an apparent competing demand, with the economic debate clearly being the stronger.

While a number of other bodies were also established by the 1970 Health Act, its most enduring contribution has been the system of health-board administration which remained largely unchanged until the late 1990s when the Eastern Regional Health Authority was established and the eastern region itself subdivided into three new health board areas. These arrangements in turn were replaced in 2005 with a more centralised set of administrative structures through the establishment of the Health Service Executive and the disbandment of the health board system.

Again considered from a public policy perspective, the structures of the health boards were interesting in that they reflected public priorities and trends of the time. For administrative purposes, each board was divided into three broad programmes, namely community care, acute hospital and special hospital services. In most health board areas the 'Programmes', which had their conceptual genesis in a business model of management, remained largely unchanged until shortly before the disbandment of the health board system.

The management and organisational structures were based on a blueprint contained in a report produced by the McKinsey and Company management consultants titled *Towards Better Healthcare Management in the Health Board*. The system was headed by a chief executive officer supported in turn by programme managers and functional officers in the management team. Somewhat ironically, at the time of its introduction, it was advocated as a system that would replace what was seen as a hierarchical system in the local health authorities. Equally ironically, the system was intended to be based on patient-care needs as opposed to geographic interests. Interestingly, this management system, purportedly based on programme delivery to specific client groups, was itself the subject of major criticism in the report *Health, the Wider Dimensions* (Department of Health, 1986). The criticisms suggested that the 'Programme' system of management was not working because it lacked integration and needed reform.

Therefore we can see that neither planning, policy formulation nor change is new in Irish health services. Neither are changes in the system of management and organisation. In fact they have gone through radical change in the latter part of the twentieth century and early part of the current century. By 1970, the government had introduced a more centralised system of healthcare administration, and in essence had assumed responsibility for the provision of a public health system that was either fully or partly subsidised through taxation (Barrington, 1987). The increasing expenditure was also commented on by Wiley (1998) who pointed out that by 1980 approximately eighty-eight per cent of health expenditure was funded through taxation and public spending. This increase in health expenditure is also confirmed by Organisation for Economic Co-operation and Development (OECD) statistics, which indicate an increase from 3.7 per cent of GDP in 1960 to 7.3 per cent in 2003 (OECD, 2003).

It is exceptionally difficult to assume that this type of investment is directly measurable in terms of outcomes, but it is at least interesting to note that the average life expectancy has increased also. In 1960 the average life expectancy at birth was seventy years, while in 2003, this had increased to seventy-eight (OECD, 2005b); infant mortality had fallen from twenty-nine to five per 1,000 live births in the same reference period (OECD, 2005c). Also of note is the fact that the density of practicing physicians (per 1,000 population) has not significantly increased from 1990 to 2003. In 1990 the density per 1,000 population was 2.2, while in 2003 it was 2.6 (OECD, 2005d) compared to an increase from 11.3 nurses to 14.8 per 1,000 in the same period (OECD, 2005e). Interestingly, nurses would claim a professional focus more related to health and caring activity than the curative focus of medicine.

In terms of lifestyle behaviours, it is also interesting to note that smoking has been the focus of ongoing attention in public policy in Ireland, culminating in a generalised ban on smoking in workplaces in 2004. While current statistics are not available, it is interesting also that the overall rate of daily smokers per 1,000 population had reduced from 45.6 to 27 per cent between 1970 and 2003 (OECD, 2005f). Unlike smoking, alcohol consumption among those over fifteen years of age increased from 4.9 litres to 13.5 litres between 1960 and 2003 (OECD, 2005g).

In terms of expenditure, the overall statistics for the period 1998–2003 are presented in Table 2.1 (on page 26). These show the increases in expenditure from the late 1990s onward. Within this total spend there is evidence of approximately a two- to threefold increase across all programmes. However, there are no statistics provided in relation to health promotion specifically. It is safe to assume that most of this expenditure relates to treatment and illness-management services. Ironically the OECD statistics demonstrate improvement in some lifestyle behaviours that in the long term should impact on service utilisation. It is difficult to gauge how this improvement might be associated with spending on health-promotion activity in the absence of published health-promotion-expenditure figures.

STRATEGIC APPROACHES AND TRENDS IN HEALTHCARE PROVISION

Kuhn (1970) argues that major paradigm shifts occur from time to time throughout history. There is little doubt that such a paradigm shift has been evident in the latter half of the twentieth century. Perhaps the most obvious shift in 'world views' becomes evident through the interconnectedness of nations, states and through the medium of technology and the technological revolution, which has resulted in the realisation of the concept of 'global village'.

Table 2.1 Estimated non-capital expenditure by programme (€m)

Programme	1998	1999	2000	2001	2002(1)	2003(2)
Community Protection Programme	99.9	136.0	224.8	314.3	275.3	298.2
Community Health Service Programme	687.2	883.5	985.0	1,191.6	1,526.1	1,611.7
Community Welfare Programme	285.5	336.5	445.9	581.4	703.8	767.6
Psychiatric Programme	347.5	394.5	433.7	497.1	563.7	612.0
Programme for the Disabled	436.6	520.8	651.6	815.9	962.9	1,122.8
General Hospital Programme	1,988.5	2,317.7	2,604.5	3,291.4	3,801.5	4,126.7
General Support Programme	194.8	218.1	264.9	318.3	333.5	388.9
Gross Total	4,040.0	4,807.3	5,610.3	7,010.1	8,166.7	8,927.8
Total non-capital income	220.9	233.4	251.3	270.8	300.2	334.3
Net total	3,819.1	4,573.9	5,359.1	6,739.3	7,866.5	8,593.5
1. Provisional 2. Outturn						

Source: Department of Health and Children (2005)

The interconnectedness and interdependence of nations has perhaps been most obvious at a global political level. In this context, conflict in the Middle East has, for example, had major repercussions and reverberations for Western societies in political, economic and social spheres of life. At the end of the twentieth century one of the more obvious forms of evidence of the 'global village' was the fact that many in Western societies were able to vicariously engage in conflicts in 'real time' as major television news networks such as Sky News and CNN as well as Arabic TV networks were able to relay images of war, conflict and atrocities virtually as they happened.

However, not all aspects of the interconnectedness of the human race are as negative as that. In terms of health and social services, the consequences of all of us being part of a greater whole is reflected in more holistic approaches to and understandings of health and healthcare. Comparisons between health services, norms, performance activity and outcomes are facilitated through the internet, with information and information sharing being also virtually instantaneous. The influence, for example, of the EU on regional and national legislation and healthcare as well as broader public policy has been enormous and increasingly the norms of healthcare models in Australia and New Zealand are being drawn upon internationally.

An interesting trend internationally in relation to health promotion is that healthcare systems have refocused to include and be dominated by issues of public health through health promotion and disease prevention. International influence and emphasis has also broadened health-service planning from its somewhat narrow traditional focus on disease management to the broader focus of health planning that incorporates health promotion and illness prevention. In an Irish context, this shift from a medically dominated model of health-service planning is perhaps most obvious and welcome in the comment of the Chief Medical Officer in his most recent report that argued that 'prevention is the cornerstone of any rational health policy' (DoHC, 2004a:5). While, as argued earlier, the emphasis on lifestyle behaviours in that report may be disappointing, it is at the very least evidence of a shift of thinking from the medical establishment that prevention (if not broader approaches to health promotion) must underpin a rational health policy.

What must be noted in an Irish context is the fact that the health and social services sector has not been short of reports and policy statements. In fact there is a long tradition of them. Examples of significant reports include those of the Commission of Inquiry on Mental Handicap which reported in 1965; the 1966 Commission of Inquiry on Mental Illness; the 1984 study group report on mental health services, titled *The Psychiatric Services: Planning for the Future*; *The Years Ahead* (Government of Ireland, 1988); *Needs and Abilities* (Government of Ireland, 1990). More recent reports include the Brennan Report and the Prospectus Report.

The vast majority of these reports and documents were important contributors to the development of services in their relevant areas. They formed the basis for service planning both at national and indeed local level in health-board areas. However, many of them were focused on providing reviews of services, performance or sector evaluations. Effectively they contributed to policy development, but at the same time were limited in that they tended to provide an overview of the desirable frameworks and operational delivery of services rather than a more strategic approach.

LEVELS AND TYPES OF PLANNING AND STRATEGY

Planning can be considered to be the most fundamental of managerial functions. Appropriate planning underpins the operations of an organisation through providing clarity in terms of the direction for the organisation. Good planning should minimise ambiguity in organisations and serve to provide evidence of leadership within the organisation. Planning should also scope an organisation in relation to its limits, thereby serving a controlling function. Planning involves the process of selecting and agreeing a vision, mission and goals for an organisation or indeed at a more micro-level for units within an organisation. Goals may of course be for a short-, medium- or long-term period and therefore will, or should, reflect the type and nature of the planning itself.

Planning within or for an organisation may happen at a variety of levels and in different forms. At a strategic level, planning should be based on an analysis of the organisation's overall environment – both external and internal, including its strengths and weaknesses. Planning should also involve the development of goals, which should ideally be based on and consistent with the mission or vision of the organisation. When these have been agreed, planning should then involve formulating a general plan of action to achieve the identified goals and allocating the appropriate resources.

Contingency planning is sometimes seen as a lower-order form of planning. This approach is also a necessary and important form of planning. However, it is problematic if this is the only form of planning in an organisation. Contingency planning involves preparing for and responding to expected, unexpected or dramatic events which can be either positive or negative in nature. Contingencies can range from natural disasters to predictable situations. These might include preparation of major emergency plans to respond to events such as a fall, an assault or strike situations. Contingency plans are not related to the overall mission or goals of the organisation. While actions are necessary to manage emergency or contingency situations, these situations are normally short-lived.

Figure 2.1 Good planning

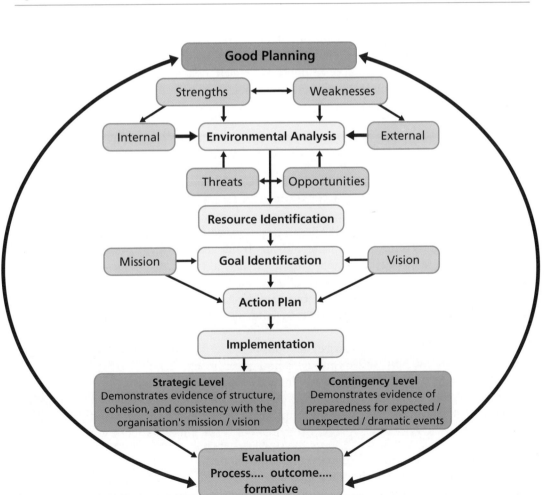

Planning, in its broadest sense, involves choosing tactics to achieve the organisation's goals. These tactics, in the context of strategic-level planning, will sustain the organisation or form the basis of its long-term wellbeing.

Strategic management is central for the development of any organisation or business. Strategic initiatives are frequently confused with policy development. However, McKevitt (1998:44) argues that strategy and strategic initiatives or actions are more comprehensive than policy statements alone. He suggests that 'strategy is concerned with the activities of service management, making explicit choices (including decisions not to do certain things), sustaining a long term commitment and maintain relationships (with clients, providers, government) in a complex environment'. As indicated, therefore, the concept of strategic planning broadly relates to the main courses of action that an organisation takes to achieve its goals. Within any organisation, the scope and complexity of strategic planning and strategy formation may vary depending on the level within the organisation at which the strategic planning takes place.

In the context of health and social planning this is an important point to remember, as there is a variety of levels of 'organisation' involved in health and social-service provision in Ireland. For example, following on the recent restructuring of health-service provision, the Health Service Executive has been delegated responsibility for public-health-service provision, while the Department of Health and Children has overall responsibility for policy decisions and directions. This has changed from a situation where eleven health boards had operational responsibility for service delivery as well as a range of voluntary and non-statutory agencies. Clearly the potential for a lack of cohesion across a wider range of providers is greater than in one organisation.

THE EVOLUTION OF A STRATEGIC PLANNING APPROACH IN THE IRISH HEALTH SYSTEM

Shaping a Healthier Future: A Strategy for Effective Healthcare in the 1990s (DoHC, 1994) was the first comprehensive national strategy to be published. While this document is frequently referred to as a health strategy, this is somewhat misleading or indeed misrepresentative of the document. This strategy argued for the restructuring of the health services within the context of a projected timeframe and outlined principles of service provision that were broadly consistent with international trends. In a review of the strategy, McAuliffe and Joyce (1998) noted that the strategy actually emerged as the result of a culmination of earlier reports that had suggested the need for radical change within both the health services and healthcare provision in Ireland. Therefore it is health service strategy, not a health strategy *per se*.

When changes in the health services are considered, it must be remembered that since the time of the Poor Law Acts, service provision and governmental action and intervention were largely concerned with and restricted to illness treatment and curative actions and focus. In keeping with international trends and evidence in the 1966 white paper referred to earlier, the concentration was on the development of medical services and hospital-based care. In fact, the term 'health services' was probably a misnomer for illness services with the service provision being largely driven by a medical model or paradigm.

Healthcare systems internationally have refocused to include and indeed perhaps to be influenced by health promotion and disease prevention, though not necessarily in that order. This change of emphasis has broadened health-service planning to adopt a more strategic stance, away from the somewhat narrow medical or illness base to a broader health-planning focus.

HEALTH PROMOTION AND PUBLIC POLICY

So, where does health promotion fit into a framework of public policy? This question needs to be addressed from at least two separate, though sometimes overlapping, perspectives. There is potentially a distinct answer to this question if we consider the 'fit' between public policy and individual practitioners in dedicated 'health promotion' functions. However, there is likely to be a different answer if we are to consider the 'fit' between a health-promotion ethos and public policy. The World Health Organization has suggested that the concept of 'healthy public policy' is characterised by 'an explicit concern for health and equity in all areas of policy and by an accountability for health impact' (WHO, 1988).

This understanding of health as opposed to illness is interesting as it raises issues of equity and accountability. It also implies inter- or cross-sectoral concern. It goes beyond the rather limiting phrase 'health policy'. The term 'healthy public policy' incorporates broader aspects of public policy than health alone. However, the term sometimes gets confused with health policy. This in turn has potential implications for the scope of practice for individual health-promotion professionals as well as health promotion as an ethos.

The notion of 'healthy public policies' and concern for them is largely based on the assumption that the broader environmental context (including the social milieu) is one of the key domains of influence on health and social status as argued in Chapter 1. Therefore concern with, as well as for, the development of 'healthy public policies' is an important component of a health-promotion ethos, and evidence of the impact of such an ethos. Governmental concern with such issues as environmental controls, agricultural standards, food production as well as processing and distribution, pollution, public transport, carbon emissions and housing policies impacts on the health and social status of individuals, groups and ultimately society. Recognition of the interrelatedness of economic and social interests is also consistent with the principles of healthy public policy. These ways of understanding health as an important contributory factor to social and economic functioning are at considerable variance with more traditional reductionist approaches.

HEALTH PROMOTION, POLITICS AND HEALTHY PUBLIC POLICY

Understanding health as an integrated resource for living highlights another key issue for health promotion, namely the political nature of health, healthy public policies and the role of health promotion in that context. Since the period following the Second World War, health has been part of the international political and social agenda. In 1948 the General Assembly of the United Nations (UN) made explicit reference to health as a universal human right when it declared that:

> Everyone has the right to a standard of living adequate for the health and well-being of himself and of his family, including food, clothing, housing and medical care and necessary social services, and the right to security in the event of unemployment, sickness, disability, widowhood, old age and other lack of livelihood in circumstances beyond his control.
>
> (United Nations 1948)

Since the Universal Declaration of Human Rights was enacted by the UN on 10 December 1948, there have been successive famines and consistent international deprivation as well as irrefutable evidence of social and economic variance in health status and opportunities internationally. This has been most notable in Third World countries, but not exclusive to them. Despite this, it has also been the case that the politics of human rights has played a prominent role in public policies and in public consciousness since that time. International debates and indeed disputes between nations over such issues as carbon emissions, environmental policies and debt reduction for Third World economies have all proved points of significant international and national debate.

Examination of the statement of this series of human rights clearly links health with social, economic and welfare rights, forming in many ways a conceptual foundation for healthy public policy and placing health within a broader policy framework. Public-health policy and health promotion in practice frequently remain somewhat narrowly focused on health and illness. We have already argued that there is a wide range of domains of influence on health status and this understanding of health and health promotion means in effect that the political nature of health promotion at international, national and local level cannot be ignored.

Harrison (2004:159) classified politics as being concerned with four key areas, as follows:
- The art of government and the activities of the state.
- The conduct and management of a community's affairs in pursuit of the notion of the (Aristotelian) 'good life'.
- The generation and resolution of conflict through compromise, negotiation and other strategies.
- The production, distribution and use of resources in the course of social existence, the nature of which is exercised through power relations.

Acceptance of this understanding of politics should indicate the relevance of political activity to health promotion – both as an ethos as well as for individual health-promotion agents. Clearly, one of the essential governmental and state functions (at least in democratic states) involves the protection and upholding of civil rights. Governmental and indeed community politics involves choice and debate. Discourse therefore becomes an essential contribution to political activity. Contribution to healthy public policy is seen as an essential component of health-promotion activity. Again drawing on Harrison's typology of political activity, politics is legitimately concerned with debate and conflict in the context of the exercise of power and the choices that societies, states or indeed local areas and services make and in the context of the power relationships that exist. It is clearly not only the right, but the responsibility of health-promotion agents to contribute to the political debates and decision-making process in the pursuit of healthy public policies.

If it is accepted that health promotion should be involved in the generation, maintenance or review of healthy public policies through political activities, a key question emerges as to the level at which this should occur and the mechanisms through which such activity should be channelled. Governmental activity is exercised at national level, but increasingly, national-level activity is at least interlinked with international levels. In a European context, the level of political activity that impacts on national political functioning has steadily increased since the inception of the European Union and its predecessor the European Economic Community. We have already identified the United Nations and the World Health Organization as key international bodies that influence national policies and politics. These and other important stakeholders are presented in Figure 2.2.

Figure 2.2 Key influences on strategy and policy formulation

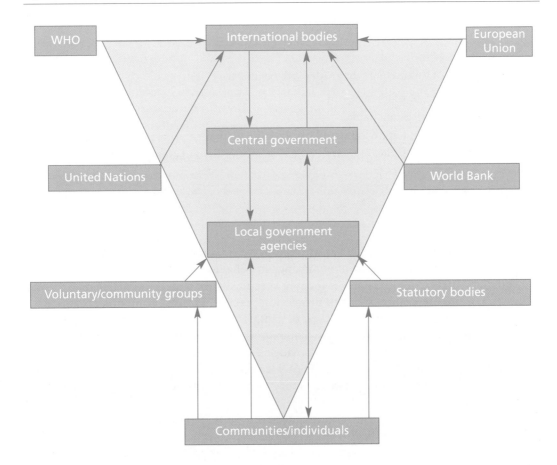

3
Health Promotion and Change Management

Learning Outcomes:

On completion of this chapter the reader will be able to:

- define the concept of change
- discuss key theories of change
- distinguish between individual and organisational change processes
- understand the relationship between health promotion and change management.

INTRODUCTION

Successful health-promotion initiatives are contingent on attention to and understanding of the processes involved in bringing about change in behaviours at individual, organisational and community levels. This chapter is focused specifically on understanding change theory, processes and their relevance to health-promotion practice. Health-promotion practitioners are concerned with influencing individual or group change or change in the organisations they work in, for example, hospitals, companies and communities. The pressure on organisations and institutions to engage in change is perhaps the most consistent pressure put upon them in recent decades (Sarason, 1996). Health-promotion professionals seek to have some influence in these change processes as they attempt to ensure organisations are health-promoting entities.

They should advocate in order to influence policy and activity among those who have power or may impact on the health of the population (Nutbeam and Harris, 2004). This should happen at either an individual or a group level. They aim to ensure that organisations or communities prioritise the promotion of health for all. Thus the health promoter operates at a number of levels in the change process. While health promotion is client-centred, it is, in essence, a political activity, in that it seeks to advocate for and influence change. All change involves compromise. This compromise may result in either loss or gain in some measure. The challenge for health promoters is to be able to support clients, communities and organisations in adjusting to the change process. The health promoter who understands organisations and who can apply appropriate strategies has a powerful tool for change (Goodman *et al.*, 2002). The same premise applies to change at community and individual level.

DEFINING CHANGE

Change can be understood as the felt or perceived differences in behaviour, circumstance or context, to the degree that the experience of the behaviour, circumstance or context is altered. Thus positive change involves a break with the traditional way of doing things towards a more effective and novel way of engaging with those same circumstances. Change may come about because we voluntarily participate or even initiate change when we are dissatisfied with the current situation, or it may be imposed upon us, for example by natural events or by those in authority.

Change may be radical, incorporating a complete overhaul of how things are done and replacement with different methods or new systems (for example the radical national restructuring of health boards to the Health Service Executive in Ireland). Or it can be small-scale, localised to solving a particular issue within an organisation. At an individual level, it may involve changing a particular behaviour such as taking more exercise or changing dietary decisions. Whether the change is radical or small-scale, managing the change process is vitally important to its success. Many change-implementation processes have failed due to lack of effective consultation with all relevant stakeholders and lack of coherent planning. Wilson (1993) has identified that all change is threatening as it brings with it much uncertainty. Given that empowerment and consultation are key principles for health-promotion practice it is imperative that health-promotion professionals endeavour to incorporate these principles into their change-planning processes.

INDIVIDUAL CHANGE

The factors that influence the success of individual change are numerous. However, the key ones relate to personal context, behaviours and attitudes. When we consider the personal context, the sense of safety that a person currently experiences becomes important. If a person is experiencing high levels of stress it is very difficult for them to make behavioural changes as the behaviour that is problematic may be a coping behaviour employed by them in dealing with that stress, for example smoking or overeating. There is also a commonly held belief that the older we become the less we embrace change. Whether or not this belief is true is debatable. However, we need to be careful not to apply generalisations to whole segments of a population. Therefore, we should be aware of this possibility but not assume it is invariably true.

The individual's current level of self-efficacy also heavily impacts upon the success of a change initiative. Bandura (1977a) offers us a succinct understanding of self-efficacy, which he defines as 'feeling certain that one can' for example, engage in and complete an action. Thus the capacity to assess self-efficacy is important in order to identify the potential for an individual to successfully implement change. Our sense of self-esteem (how we feel about or perceive ourselves) influences how we understand ourselves and how we believe others may perceive us. If we feel good about ourselves it is easier to embrace a change.

However, if we feel a sense of failure with regard to ourselves then it becomes more difficult to motivate ourselves and/or successfully initiate and maintain a change in behaviour. In other words, the belief that we can or cannot change transposes itself into a self-fulfilling prophecy. Thus the health promoter needs to be aware that when they are working at an individual level it is not simply a matter of outlining the change necessary and expecting that the client can engage with the change without support. The health promoter must work *with* the client in order to assess and facilitate the enhancement of an individual's sense of self-efficacy with regard to change. They also need to examine with the client their home, work and social environments to identify the supportive and hindering factors in order to generate strategies, to incorporate supports and to minimise threats to the success of the change endeavour.

A number of individual behavioural change approaches have been set out as effective models for health-promotion practice. A simplistic approach to understanding behavioural change would be to assume that the giving of relevant information leads to a change in attitude, then in behaviour, leading to improved health. However, this assumption is overly simplistic in nature. This understanding mistakenly assumes that there is a direct correlation between information-giving and behavioural change. Behaviour is more directly influenced by our attitudes and beliefs, which are deeply held. Attitudes and beliefs are most influential with regard to motivation and demotivation in behavioural change. Therefore, models of change that incorporate an understanding of the processes and cycles in behaviour change as well as the role of attitudes, beliefs, self-efficacy, self-esteem, social norms and the role of significant others (such as peers and family) are necessary in order to build a comprehensive understanding of the complexity of behavioural change.

Health belief model

The health belief model is probably the most widely subscribed to in that it is relied upon in order to arrive at some understanding of the reasons behind the health decisions that individuals make. This model was first suggested by Hochbaum (1958) but was later much further developed by Rosenstock (1966, 1974) and Becker (1984).

The health belief model has its origins in illness-prevention approaches (Finfgeld *et al.*, 2003). It originally sought to understand the reasons why individuals who were at risk of disease or illness would not participate in preventative efforts or screening programmes. The health belief model essentially suggests that when a number of conditions converge, an individual who is susceptible to illness is likely to take action. These conditions relate to perceptions of the seriousness of the disease or illness, perceived barriers to the action taken, as well as the 'cue' to take a 'health action' (Wai *et al.*, 2005).

However, another key element of the health belief model relates to the concept of self-efficacy. Self-efficacy essentially relates to the belief of an individual in their capacity to undertake the action necessary to address the health issue concerned. The model draws heavily on the understanding that people's decisions with regard to engaging in behavioural change are influenced by the sense that they can successfully effect the change (self-efficacy). The health belief model also acknowledges that there is a range of demographic, psychosocial and individual factors that may indirectly influence health behaviours.

What is also influential is the belief that the benefits of the change far outweigh the costs. In other words that the desired outcome is worth the engagement and effort. For an individual to be motivated to change their behaviour, it must cause some potential discomfort either currently or potentially in the near future. The change must be salient (needed) and the individual must feel competent to successfully complete the change.

Tones and Green (2004) identify four major beliefs relevant to the health belief model. The first is that the individual must feel personal susceptibility to the negative event (illness). The second is the belief that the event is serious and threatens the existing status quo. The third is that the proposed change will be effective in reducing the threat from the event, and finally that the proposed change will not have too great a cost. According to Tones and Green (2004:81) two later important additions to the model are the concepts of cues to action and health motivation. Along with the four beliefs outlined, a 'jolt into action' or trigger may also be needed to embark on the change (cue to action) and an understanding of the health motivation also aids the explanatory value of the health belief model. In other words people do not engage in change action unless they feel motivated to do so by the belief that illness is a real possibility for them, or if they believe the change would not work.

Critics of the health belief model have argued that it is limited in that it can account for the variance in individuals' health behaviours that are linked to attitudes and beliefs but the model does not take into account other influences on behaviour such as social, environmental and economic factors (Janz and Becker, 1984). The health belief model has been found to be most useful when it is used for the preventative behaviours for which it was developed, such as screening and immunisation. However, it is perceived to be less useful in areas of complex and long-term behavioural issues such as alcohol and tobacco use (Nutbeam and Harris, 2004). Its usefulness is in the recognition of the importance of attitudes and beliefs as a central reference point in the promotion of individual behavioural change.

Theory of reasoned action

The theory of reasoned action is attributed to Ajzen and Fishbein (1980) and this theory differs from the health belief model in that it makes explicit the link between an individual's attitudes and their subsequent behaviours. Within this model it is proposed that a person's behaviour is heavily influenced by their intentions which themselves are heavily influenced by attitudes. Ajzen and Fishbein (1980) argue that behaviour is governed by two main influences: that of a belief (for example, exercise can benefit my health status) and the degree of positive or negative association with that belief. For example if the belief is positively and strongly held then it will more than likely influence behaviour (Bennett and Hodgson, 1992).

The second significant influence is the impact of subjective norms on the decision-making of an individual. In other words the influence of what significant others (such as peers and family, even on occasion celebrities) will think of their decision. The strength of the belief held and the influence of the subjective norms combine to form an intention for an individual. The influence of the subjective norm can be a positive motivator. For example, being in a social group with those who do not drink alcohol to excess can mean an individual may be less inclined to become drunk. However, the opposite may also be true. Where a drink culture permeates, an individual may be less inhibited about being drunk. Therefore health-promotion professionals wishing to support the individual behavioural change process and working within this model need to examine the stability of the beliefs held, how long such beliefs are held and the influence of significant others in contributing to or reinforcing such behaviour.

Ajzen and Fishbein also further develop this model to include the degree of perceived control in influencing intention. They argue that if a person feels they have control over their behaviour, then they are more likely to engage in the behavioural change. Thus Ajzen and Fishbein advocate changing the title of their model to the Theory of Planned Behaviour as a development of the theory of reasoned action alone (Ajzen and Fishbein, 1980).

Stages of change model

The stages of change model, also referred to as the transtheoretical model, was originally developed within psychotherapy as an attempt to synthesise an approach to therapeutic engagement and to make sense of the wide variety of psychotherapeutic approaches (Prochaska, 1979). The term 'transtheoretical' therefore denotes the fact that this theory incorporates many theories of change. The analysis of the theories (hence the title 'transtheoretical') resulted in the identification of ten 'common' mechanisms or stages taken to arrive at a decision to adopt new behaviours or facilitate change. These were referred to as change processes and included the activities and processes presented in Table 3.1.

The model itself emerged over time (Prochaska and DiClemente, 1983) and is essentially concerned with the structure or stages and processes underlying intentional change. While the model was originally developed in relation to problem behaviours, it has since been used to sitive health-related behaviours are acquired (Houlihan, 1999). In essence, ...es a combination and continuum of cognitive and behavioural processes ...ove through, from a position of unwillingness or lack of awareness for the ...ange behaviours, through to the situation where changes are engaged in and ...aintained across time. It would be incorrect to suggest that change through each of the stages is sequential or linear, even though this was the original assumption.

Prochaska and DiClemente's model (1986) helps practitioners support individuals in successfully engaging with the change process. A central belief that permeates the stages of change model is that behaviour change is complex and is a process rather than an event (Xiao et al., 2004). In fact, Prochaska et al. argue that change occurs more frequently in a spiral fashion, with change backward and forward possible and individualistic in nature (Prochaska et al., 1992). They note that where individuals change, that process is not necessarily ordered or indeed consistently maintained. Core to successful implementation of the stages of change model is attention to individual readiness and preparedness to engage in the change process, as the level of motivation and preparedness deeply impacts on the success of the change endeavour.

Table 3.1 Change process

Change process	Definition of change process
Consciousness raising	Finding and learning new facts, ideas and tips that support the healthy behaviour change
Social liberation	Realising that the social norms are changing in the direction of supporting the healthy behaviour change
Dramatic relief	Experiencing the negative emotions that go along with unhealthy behaviour risks
Self re-evaluation	Realising that the behaviour change is an important part of one's identity as a person
Self liberation	Making a firm commitment to change
Counter conditioning	Substituting healthy alternative behaviour and cognition for the unhealthy behaviour
Stimulus control	Removing reminders or cues to engage in the unhealthy behaviour
Contingency management	Increasing the rewards for the positive behaviour change and decreasing the rewards for the unhealthy behaviour
Helping relationships	Seeking and using social support for the healthy behaviour change
Environmental re-evaluation	Realising the negative impact of the unhealthy behaviour or the positive impact of the healthy behaviour on one's personal, social and physical environment

Source: Prochaska *et al.*, 1996

The stages of change model is represented as cyclical in nature and incorporating five stages. The first stage is identified as *precontemplation*. This stage of the cycle represents an individual who has not even thought about the problems with the given behaviour (for example, smoking) and therefore is not engaged in any cognitive process with regard to individual change. With regard to an example such as smoking or alcohol use, it is difficult to imagine that any individual is unaware of the problems associated with such behaviours and their ensuing impact on individual health. So at this precontemplation stage it may be that the person is aware of the potential harm of the behaviour but is not contemplating addressing that behaviour as yet.

The second stage of the model is *contemplation*. This is the stage in which the individual considers making a specific change to their behaviour. This contemplation may be prompted by a health concern. For example, someone with a medical condition such as high cholesterol may contemplate engaging in more exercise or losing weight as a result of their GP's advice. Alternatively the contemplation may come from motivation within the individual himself or herself. Where the impetus comes from is not the central issue, what is important are the supports the individual may put in place so that they may implement their change successfully.

The third stage is *preparation*. This is the stage where the individual looks at the practical implications of what the behavioural change will mean for them and what types of supports they will need to put in place in order to successfully implement their change. For example, for a reduction of alcohol intake a person may need to decide to no longer engage in 'round' buying in a pub and may need to change their habits with regard to frequenting the pub. They may decide, perhaps, to go to the pub later in the evening for one or two drinks before closing, or to go just once a week. If the change is with regard to smoking, they may initially need to avoid the stimulus that encourages their smoking (for example, coffee with friends) until they feel confident that they may decline to smoke. Perhaps they may need to inform their friends of their planned change in order to gain peer support. The preparation stage is important as many individuals take to their change initiative very well for the first week or two but the motivation can wane very easily as time and the immediate reason behind the impetus passes. Therefore, putting in place the relevant supports is key to successful implementation of change.

The fourth stage of the transtheoretical model of change is the *action* stage. This is the stage where the individual actually implements their change. This stage is frequently attempted with much effort and motivation. It is important that the approach is level and commensurate with the individual's lifestyle so that it becomes a change that can be maintained with relative ease.

The fifth stage in this model is identified as *maintenance*. This is where the action of change has become integrated into the individual's life and is now part of their lifestyle behaviours. In the planning of the change maintenance is planned for so that integration of the change is a core aspect of the change process.

While the duration of each stage will be very personal and individuals may move in a spiral fashion through the stages and between them (in both directions), the proposition is that the stages themselves are consistent.

The stages of change or transtheoretical model also proposes a relationship between the processes and the stages of change. These are presented in Table 3.2.

ges of change

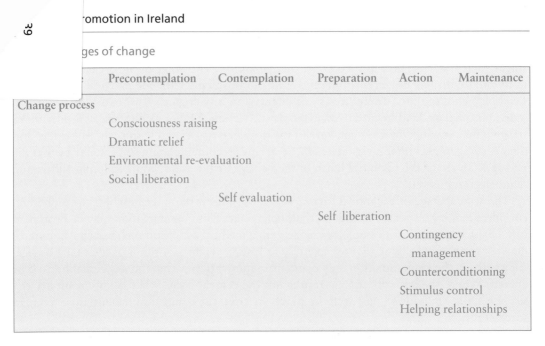

	Precontemplation	Contemplation	Preparation	Action	Maintenance
Change process					
	Consciousness raising				
	Dramatic relief				
	Environmental re-evaluation				
	Social liberation				
		Self evaluation			
			Self liberation		
				Contingency management	
				Counterconditioning	
				Stimulus control	
				Helping relationships	

Source: Prochaska *et al.*, 1996

Relapse is also a possibility during the stage of change cycle. It is estimated that an individual may commence and engage in various elements of the cycle of change approximately three times if not more in an attempt to change some deeply ingrained behaviours. It is imperative that health-promotion practitioners do not hold a blame approach to the relapse stage, as it is a normal part of any change process. Deeply ingrained norms of behaviour and attitude are particularly difficult to change. In supporting the individual in surmounting the relapse stage, the practitioner should remind the individual of the popular maxim that it is no 'sin' to fall, but it is to lie there. Individuals should be encouraged to believe that they can participate in their own rescue and that change is very much possible for them no matter how seemingly difficult.

The transtheoretical or stages of change model has much to offer health-promotion practitioners and indeed has become an integral aspect of behavioural-change promotion. It provides a framework for understanding as well as influencing change. Its strength lies in the motivation of individuals to take charge of their own change process as well as helping to discover the individual's readiness to engage with the change process. If the readiness is weak then the practitioner needs to spend time supporting the individual in contemplating and planning their change initiative. Therefore, the key role of the health-promotion agent is to match the stage at which the individual is on the cycle with the intervention, rather than making the individual fit the intervention. Imposing the order of change is the least successful of all change initiatives. Understanding the processes as well as the stages of change contributes (or at least potentially contributes) to health-promotion agents' operations either at an individual or a community level in terms of influencing health-related decisions or lifestyle choices.

Social learning theory or social cognition theory

Social cognition theory has its roots in social learning theory and is most heavily influenced by Bandura's work (1977b, 1986, 1995). Social learning theory is predicated on the understanding that we learn through our processes of socialisation and that as individuals we can never be divorced from the influence of our environment and socialisation.

Bandura argues that the relationship between an individual and their environment is deeply complex and evolutionary in nature. A key mode of learning by individuals is vicarious learning through the modelling and influence of those within their environment. For example, in a workplace where many people do not like smoking, an individual may become less inclined to smoke as it is considered a socially unacceptable behaviour. Bandura terms this relationship 'reciprocal determinism', where the individual, their environment and their behaviour continuously interact and influence each other (Nutbeam and Harris, 2004:20). Often the influence of such informal assertions or interactions can become mainstream within a society; an example would be the smoking ban in workplaces in Ireland in 2004.

Bandura also argues that in addition to reciprocal determinism, personal cognitive processes are necessary for and influence behavioural change. Vicarious learning or learning through observing the behaviours of others is influential in behavioural change. For example, where people see the benefits of healthy diet and exercise in others and these emerge as socially valued behaviours, they may decide to engage in similar behaviour. While the value we as individuals place on behaviour is important in influencing change, the social influence and consequence of behaviour modelling is a significant element to be considered within this model. In addition self-efficacy or the belief we have in our capacity to complete an action is deeply influential with regard to our intentions to engage in behavioural change.

What becomes evident with regard to Bandura's social cognitive model is the complexity of factors that influence human behaviour and particularly behavioural change processes. For successful behavioural change, an individual must be supported in exploring the implications of their proposed change from the perspective of their sense of efficacy with regard to completing the action. In addition, it is important to examine the impact of the change on their relationship with significant others and their interaction with their social environment. Thus, a health-promotion professional operating within this model is arguably less interventionist than in other health-promotion models and rather takes on the role of change agent 'facilitating change through modification of the social environment and the development of personal competencies that enable individuals to act to improve their health' (Nutbeam and Harris, 2004:22).

In practice, most practitioners do not rely on a single model, but in fact adopt an eclectic approach, whereby they draw on the range of models already described. The chosen approach must provide the best support for their clients who are embarking on change and practitioners must be able to base the rationale for their choice on sound theoretical underpinnings. The following prerequisites for individual change must be considered in the selection of approach. The reason for change may be brought to the fore due to some illness or potential illness but the *desire* for change must be self-initiated. Imposed change is rarely if ever successful. The behaviour must be salient to the person and the salience or importance must be long-term.

A commonly held belief within health-promotion practice is that the behaviour under change must not be part of an individual's coping strategies. However, we contend that this is not necessarily possible. For example, where an individual uses smoking behaviour as a coping strategy to manage stress, this behaviour must be addressed appropriately. We believe that it is morally imperative that smoking be addressed and the individual supported in developing more positively adaptive coping responses. Ethical practice in healthcare demands this. In that context, much time must be spent in support-planning for alternative behaviour strategies, which can be many and varied to provide an appropriate repertoire of behaviours which will maintain interest. To do this, the change agent must identify and make available as many social supports as possible. Finally, in doing so, they should also facilitate their clients in creating their own network of social support.

Brief interventions model

The brief interventions model of behavioural change is regularly used by health-promotion practitioners in support of clients who are attempting to embark on some form of behavioural change. It is well contested and critics of the model argue that there is no evidence of long-term effectiveness of the brief interventions approach. Proponents of brief interventions argue strongly for the skills development and capacity building it provides for health-promotion practitioners and those they train in the skills of brief interventions. In some geographical regions of Ireland brief intervention currently enjoys some popularity among health-promotion professionals. It is encouraged as an effective skills-development initiative in response to the need for behavioural change strategies, with specific reference to smoking, alcohol use, nutrition, physical activity and sexual health.

The Brief Interventions Skills for Health Promotion programme was developed by Barbara Wren and Karen Thomas in 2001. The programme is skills-based and is founded entirely on the stages of change model for behaviour change. The programme functions by paying particular attention to the processes that underpin change and emphasises the skills and strategies that are needed for the promotion of health-behaviour change (Wren and Thomas, 2001:2).

A programme such as brief interventions functions as a five-day training plan. It is carried out with health and social-care professionals in their local areas. It is designed for ease of dissemination and skills development so that those trained in the skills of brief interventions will be able to successfully initiate a process of change for clients or friends. These clients or friends may currently be engaging in behaviour that may threaten their health status such as smoking or excessive alcohol use. Those skilled in brief interventions are able to identify the individual's current stage on the stages of change cycle and adopt an intervention appropriate to that stage. For example, if an individual is at the contemplation stage with regard to their behaviour the techniques would be to offer support, to complete a decisional balance (weigh up the pros and cons of the change), identify potential barriers to change and discuss concerns. The brief interventions course is focused on the skills needed to initiate and support change; it does not explore medical implications of behaviour.

ORGANISATIONAL CHANGE

Kurt Lewin's unfreezing/freezing model

Lewin (1958) advocated a three-stage approach to change with specific reference to organisations. A key assumption that influences his understanding of organisational behaviour is that traditions become embedded or frozen into place. In order to engage in change, there are three phases that must be followed. The first is a process of *unfreezing* the status quo. This stage incorporates the introduction of the need for change. An examination of the factors currently in place and of the factors needed to influence the process of change is undertaken. Often strategies to raise awareness are engaged in at this stage. For example, the introduction of an educative programme, development of communication strategies needed to support the change and dissemination of information can be embarked upon. Frequently key personnel are targeted to enlist their support in order to persuade others to adopt the proposed change.

The second stage is the *change* itself. At this stage the organisation is actively developing and engaging in the new behaviours they wish to adopt. They are also adopting new attitudes and values with regard to the change being experienced. This is followed by the third stage, referred to as the *refreezing* stage. This occurs once people become used to the change and it becomes embedded in the organisation. When this has happened, it effectively means that the change has been consolidated, ensuring it continues. The aim at this stage is to ensure that systems of information dissemination and communication are in place to facilitate the embedding of the new change into the mission, values and culture of the organisation. Lewin's three-stage approach to organisational change has been particularly influential in change theory and has been expanded upon and developed by many other theorists. It remains a core strategy in many change-implementation processes in organisations globally.

Force field analysis

Central to Lewin's three-stage approach to organisational change is the concept which has become known as force field analysis. Lewin was heavily influenced by the laws of natural science and physics in particular. He believed that each action has an equal and opposite reaction as set out by the fundamental laws of physics. In applying this to organisational behaviour, Lewin (1951) argued that in a given situation there are enabling (driving) and diabling (restraining) forces. They act in opposition to each other to maintain the status quo. Lewin warned that if one simply increased driving forces in order to forge ahead with a change intervention, one in fact does little to change the equilibrium as the level of opposition simply increases as well. Only increasing driving forces results in exactly the same situation which is now existing under increased tension and pressure.

In order to effect a change one must overcome the restraining forces by spending time reducing resistance before and during the change implementation. If a change agent has not examined the restraining forces prior to implementing a change, it is likely that the restraining forces (which will strengthen when challenged) will (if not immediately, then within a short time) bring about a reversion to the status quo. Clearly the implication for change in organisations is the need for close attention to the diffusion of resistance before embarking on a change process. Thus an effective health-promotion professional acting as a change agent will engage in a force field analysis. In other words they will examine the restraining and enabling forces and create a strategy to strengthen the enabling forces and decrease the restraining ones in order to embed the change in the organisation. Lewin argued that an effective way to do this is to focus some attention on the organisational culture and subjective norms that predominate and function to maintain the status quo.

Figure 3.1 Lewin's force field analysis

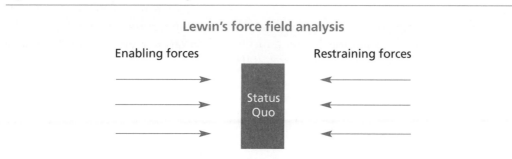

Diffusion of innovations theory

While individual behavioural change is a central focus of health-promotion work, so too is change specific to organisations and communities. Within organisations and communities the development of policies and strategies that are conducive to the promotion of health are central to creating healthy environments as prioritised by the Ottawa Charter (WHO, 1986). 'Understanding the ways in which social structures impact on health and developing skills in working with communities is important in contemporary health promotion practice' (Nutbeam and Harris, 2004:26). Diffusion of innovation theory (Rogers, 1983) has become a popular approach in health-promotion practice in order to effectively disseminate new ideas and strategies within communities.

By innovation, Rogers means an idea or way of working that is perceived as new or novel. Diffusion means how the innovation is communicated and disseminated throughout a community. Thus in health promotion a diffusion of innovations approach would be specific to how a new health-related strategy or behaviour is disseminated throughout a community. This would include the types of communication channels employed to facilitate the diffusion.

Rogers argues that people approach change very differently. Within any community there are what he terms innovators. These are the initial small number of individuals who immediately take on the change. He cautions, however, that these might not have the staying power to remain with the initiative for long periods of time. Therefore, while these innovators are very important in gaining an initial foothold for the innovation, they must be quickly followed with more individuals who come on board. Innovators serve an important function in that they contribute to awareness raising for the innovation.

Early adopters are those within the community who subsequently commit to supporting the innovation. Rogers warns of the importance of bringing these early adopters on board, as they will pioneer the innovation. As soon as others within the community can see the benefits and potential of the change process they will then come on-stream. These late converts to the innovation are referred to as the late majority. As with any change process, some may not engage with the change process at all but in diffusions of innovations approaches this is a very small minority.

Rogers offers some key insights into the change process within communities which are also applicable to organisational change. Central to this theory is the identification of opinion leaders. Health-promotion professionals hoping to foster an effective change process within a community or organisation must spend time identifying key personnel who are influential opinion leaders. These individuals will influence the uptake of the health behaviours that health-promotion agents are attempting to promote. The health-promotion change agent will explore the dynamics of the opinion leadership in order to be able to incorporate it into the their change process.

Rogers identifies the tactical importance of the change agent as someone who can effectively strategise in order to bring as many members of the community or organisation on board with the innovation as possible. The change agent can act as role model or identify role models in order to support the change process. There are similarities with Bandura's social cognitive model in that vicarious learning through observation and role modelling is an aspect of both theories (Nutbeam and Harris, 2004).

Action planning

As with any change process creating an effective action plan is central to the success of change implementation. It is the lack of time spent on the planning stage that regularly results in the failure of change-implementation processes. In planning, a change agent should be attempting to answer questions such as:

- What are the specific needs of the target group?
- What are my goals? (What am I trying to achieve?)
- What are my specific objectives or targets?
- How do I ensure that my change plan is consultative and collaborative in nature?
- How will I evidence what has been done?

Needs assessment

Once a general area of change has been identified, it is imperative that an effective needs-assessment process is undertaken. It is strongly recommended that the needs-assessment process be consultative in nature from as early a stage as possible. Needs assessments are often carried out without examining what types of needs-assessment processes those about to be affected by the change perceive as worthwhile and valuable for them. These assessments are frequently carried out by external change agents or by someone in the organisation who is divorced somewhat from the general population of the organisation – frequently by position of hierarchical authority.

A process of backward mapping (Elmore, 1989) is the most effective way of ensuring a relevant and successful change-implementation process. Elmore argues strongly that those closest to the point of change are best positioned to inform change agents of what changes are necessary and also of the most successful strategies the change agent might employ. This differs from 'top-down approaches' to change management in which normative change processes are engaged in, leaving those affected by the change disempowered in the process. In these types of situation, those most affected have no voice in planning a process that impacts upon their working life. Normative needs are those defined by the professional or expert according to their perception. Normative needs assessments are disempowering and a process of backward mapping from the earliest stage of needs assessment is necessary so that even the research design specific to needs assessment is consultative in nature.

Needs assessments can be conducted in a variety of ways and the consultation process with those whose needs are being assessed means that change-agent or researcher bias does not predominate in the design of the needs-assessment tools. Certain needs within an organisation may already be widely articulated. These can be recorded and included in a needs-assessment report. Examples might include such concerns as numbers of clients, recruitment and retention issues (if there are not enough staff to deal with clients), space, environmental matters or general need for refurbishment in the organisation. Other needs are not so easily expressed but are felt and therefore a research instrument may be the best way of tapping into those needs. These might be identified through a questionnaire, the use of focus groups or interviews, with anonymity guaranteed in the reporting of data. In relation to illness, epidemiological data may be available and can be incorporated in a needs-assessment report. The first priority is to set the scope for the needs assessment so that the process is focused, relevant and specific.

Once the needs assessment is completed and needs are identified they must be prioritised. Some key questions that can aid this process are:

- What type of need is identified? (Is it felt, expressed or normative?)
- Who is the need most pertinent for?
- Is the need within the scope of the change proposed?
- Is it a realistic proposition to address this need? (Can it be successfully addressed?)

Setting aims and objectives

Once the needs assessment has been conducted and the needs prioritised, the next stage of the process is the setting of aims and specific objectives or outcomes for the change implementation. Aims are the general goal or area of focus, for example in a workplace health-promotion change initiative a general aim might be to increase levels of awareness with regard to healthy eating at work. Objectives are more specific and are more tightly measurable. It is recommended that objectives are SMART, in other words that they are Specific, Measurable, Attainable, Realistic and Timely. Therefore in the same workplace initiative, an objective might be to make healthy options available in the canteen in order to encourage healthy eating. Another may be to have a specific awareness campaign implemented in all sections of the workplace. In planning aims and objectives it is worth noting that the objectives should fulfil the general aims. A rule of thumb we recommend to help in this process is to think of the aim as generally where you want to go (the destination) and to think of the objectives as specifically how you plan to get there (the map).

Achieving the aims and objectives

So far we have addressed the needs assessment, the prioritising of needs and the setting of the aims and objectives. The next stage in the action plan is the method of implementation. In change planning, the processes of change engaged in are very important to the success of the endeavour. The methods or strategies that will best fulfil the objectives in a manner that is consultative and empowering for those affected by the change are what must be prioritised. It is helpful at this stage of the planning to have identified key stakeholders who may act as opinion leaders and support the change. Also any resources that may be useful need to be identified.

The change agent is an effective resource in themselves, as are individuals who may be able to support the change. A useful external resource may be found in the local health-promotion unit, which is likely to have personnel with expertise in the area of change proposed. A SWOT analysis that identifies the Strengths, Weakness, Threats and Opportunities of the organisation or community with whom the change agent is working can often be an effective means for identifying support and potential stumbling blocks for the change.

Evaluation

Any change process must incorporate an evaluation procedure from the outset. Evaluation means placing value on what has been done and making judgments with regard to the quality of the initiative. Evidence-based practice is an important aspect of any health promoter's work and evaluation is one way of being able to evidence the quality and scope of work being conducted. We suggest that evaluation is approached from two perspectives, namely *process* and *outcome* evaluation. *Process evaluation* looks at the process by which the change was implemented and should occur throughout the change initiative. Reports from the evaluation should be given at strategic intervals to key stakeholders, so that the evaluation can be *formative* in nature. If an issue emerges from the ongoing evaluation it can be addressed during the change implementation and therefore it is not left until the end when little can be done to rectify the situation for the current change. *Outcome* evaluation then measures whether the objectives have been achieved and whether the change implementation can be claimed as a successful endeavour.

Some practitioners choose to adopt an action-research approach to evaluating their work.

Action research is an effective strategy that can be used by a change agent to monitor their practice in order to improve it. The principles of emancipation, empowerment and consultation that are central to action research are also commensurate with health-promotion practice.

Evaluation of change implementation is important so that practitioners can improve their practice as change agents, so that the resources used can be accounted for. In addition, evaluation, in which the success of the endeavour can be evidenced, can aid in the bid for funding to continue such work within a community or organisation.

Reducing resistance to change

It is fair to say that most people are unsure about change. Therefore, the implementation of change requires much attention to the diffusion of potential resistances. Even change which will improve people's health status may be met with resistance, despite the obvious long-term benefits that are associated with engaging with the change. Hussey (1995) identifies factors that can cause resistance to change. These are listed as actual threats that may affect an individual's identity or status such as threatened demotion or additional workloads. They also include imposed change that is forced upon individuals and a lack of belief or trust in those implementing the change.

If the principles of health promotion, such as empowerment and consultation, are adhered to, many of these resistances will be diffused throughout the modelling of the change process itself. Transparent communication processes, in which all members of the organisation feel they are aware of the processes engaged in, diffuses the rumour mill and avoids potential stumbling blocks. Thus health-promotion practitioners who embody the principles of empowerment and transparency in their consultative processes should be able to incorporate these principles easily into their work as change agents.

4
Health Promotion and Empowerment

Learning Outcomes:

On completion of this chapter the reader will be able to:

- define the concept of empowerment
- discuss the centrality of power to empowerment
- debate issues relating to client and practitioner empowerment
- understand the concept of social capital and its relevance to health
- debate the processes associated with community development within the context of empowerment.

EMPOWERMENT

Empowerment is a term widely used in health-promotion theory and practice. Health-promotion practitioners are called upon to work with clients in a manner which fosters their capacity to engage in action and to become both self-reliant and self-motivated with regard to behavioural change. Therefore, an expert-driven approach to heath promotion is not commensurate with the values of empowerment, which is a central tenet of health promotion and should also underpin all practice. Many assumptions prevail with regard to empowerment, such as the belief that one person can empower another or even that empowerment is a given in any health-promoting practice. However, a critical analysis of empowerment as a value and a process offers a very different picture.

Traditional definitions of health have been expanded from focusing only on physical and psychological health to the inclusion of a sense of general wellbeing.

> Physical and so-called 'mental' health, are inextricably intertwined with well being: the enjoyment of a life of quality in terms of feeling good, in terms of decent housing and enough to eat and wear, in terms of being a valued member of families and communities and also in terms of being without pain, fear and anger.
>
> (McCubbin, 2001)

In addition to these criteria we would argue that a sense of wellbeing is dependent on a sense of control and power with regard to one's capacity to engage in decision-making for areas that affect one's own life and health. Supporting people in taking control of their decision-making processes and in becoming able to effectively advocate for their own lives is often referred to as empowerment. Empowerment is central in the Ottawa Charter's definition of health promotion as 'the process of enabling people to increase control over and improve their health' (WHO, 1986).

DEFINING EMPOWERMENT

Empowerment has been defined in different ways. Rappaport, Swift and Hess (1984) see empowerment as a process by which people, organisations and communities gain mastery over their own lives. Torre (1986) also deems empowerment as a process but one in which people become strong enough to participate in, share in the control of and influence events and institutions affecting their lives. Being able to influence factors that affect one's life is considered important to empowerment. Wallerstein (1992) argues that empowerment is a multi-level concept that involves people taking control and mastery over their lives in the context of their social environment. Central to all these definitions so far is the sense of mastery and control that is fostered within an individual, organisation or a community. A sense of control is a key facet of empowerment and authors such as Freire (1970) broaden the definition to incorporate a sense of social justice when he argues that empowerment is a social-action process which promotes participation of people, organisations and communities towards the goals of increased individual and community control, political efficacy, improved quality of life and social justice.

This theme of 'process' is also evident in other definitions. For example, Jackson *et al.* (1996) equally place heavy emphasis on the continuing process element of empowerment and also identify that those who help in the empowerment process build on already existing strengths within the networks of the client and community.

> Empowerment is an ongoing process of enabling individuals, families, groups or communities to increase and/or maintain control over their lives and environments through independent decision making, achievement of their goals and a belief in their own power and self worth. Those assisting in this process build on existing strengths of the individual, family, group or community and facilitate the recognition of internal and external power/resources available for goal attainment.
>
> (Jackson *et al.*, 1986:7)

Empowerment can also be understood as a state of being as well as a process that is encouraged through collective participation in order to make changes with regard to self, organisation and community (Mason, 1993). What is of interest in Mason's work is that personal competence with regard to knowledge and the formulation of action plans to achieve individual and collective goals is also considered an essential medium through which the process is achieved.

Care is needed in the approach and understanding that we adopt towards empowerment in health promotion. The term empowerment is bandied about so frequently without substance that it has become perceived as a buzzword that appears to deal with unlimited facets of relationships between practitioners, clients and communities. Carey (2000:28) warns that empowerment has become 'the universal cure-all for all the ills of the post industrial age'. In health promotion the term empowerment is used frequently to denote the type of relationships practitioners attempt to adopt with clients or communities, often without any critical realisation of what exactly this means for health-promotion practice. Despite the popularity of the usage of empowerment as a strategy and an ideology there exists little coherent understanding of what constitutes empowerment. Therefore the place to begin in creating a coherent understanding is with power itself, as it is the central premise upon which empowerment is based.

Power

The concept of power is central to all definitions of empowerment and is implicit within the relationship between the health-promotion practitioner and their clients. In order to arrive at a comprehensive and pragmatic vision of empowerment a critical analysis of how we understand power is necessary. The role of power within our daily lives, within our structures and relationships is not something we hold up for critical analysis very often and we regularly assume that power has no impact on our health or on health-services provision. We can mistakenly assume that it is more relevant in the realm of governmental politics.

However, power influences all aspects of health and our health service. An illustrative example would be to ask the question, Where is the relative power distributed within the mental health services? Is the locus of control and power with the patients? With the family members? With the health professionals? With the drug companies? With those in administration who influence policy or with government officials? The client is the least powerful in such situations. The interests of the 'psychosocially distressed or distressing persons who become labelled with mental illness are likely to be the last to be met' (McCubbin, 2001:77).

Clients often tend to be marginalised within the experience of illness as they generally don't have access to the nomenclature (i.e. language and terminology) that medical professionals such as doctors or nurses may use while engaging in their treatment. Their sense of control over their level of knowledge is heavily dependent on the time spent in clarification by the health professional. Clients can feel alienated by the label of their illness, such as cancer or schizophrenia. They often do not feel that they have personal power to make decisions about their care and rely heavily on the advice of the health professional they are dealing with. As the healthcare expert generally determines what actions to take and as it is usually in the clients' interest to adhere to their recommendations they regularly feel they have no power or choice with regard to their healthcare (Menon, 2002). In this context, therefore, it is of great importance that the practitioner foster relationships with clients that are cognisant of the possible alienation the client may feel. Practitioners must endeavour to create relationships that encourage clients to be actively involved in their care.

Power is manifested in a variety of different guises. Tones and Green (2004) offer a succinct outline of the most prominent manifestations of power particularly relevant to health promotion. *Legitimate power* is bestowed by a given social system or is structurally invested in a given system. An example of this is the power vested in monolithic institutions such as a national healthcare system or a national education system. *Expert power* is evident in the perceived expertise of individuals or organisations. *Reward power* is based on an organisation's or individual's capacity to bestow reward. *Coercive power* is evident in an individual's capacity to create and apply sanctions. *Referent power* can be perceived in an individual's capacity to influence, based on other individuals' willingness to be influenced.

While all these manifestations of power are relevant to discourses of power and control, expert power is the one most relevant for a specific discourse of empowerment in healthcare. Within an understanding of expert power, knowledge becomes equated with power. This argument is central to the work of Foucault (1997), who is perhaps the most influential theorist with regard to power. A core premise that permeates all of his work is that power and knowledge are inextricably linked. He argues, in his critique of the medical profession, that the centralisation of knowledge within the preserve of elite experts such as the medical practitioner reinforces structural forms of power and domination. This serves to create alienation for clients and service users who do not possess the knowledge nor the nomenclature necessary to access services on an equitable basis. Foucault's work has significant relevance for discourses specific to the approach used by health-promotion professionals who, if they adhere to the spirit of Ottawa, will reject an expert-driven approach for a more client-centred and empowering one.

Foucault (1997) advocates that rather than perceiving power as an objective entity or construct, it is more accurate to understand power as distributed throughout social networks or as actively constructed in the relationships that people engage in on a daily basis. This reconceptualisation challenges us to understand power as constituted in the relationships we have with others. It further challenges health-promotion practitioners to ask such critical questions as:

- How do we understand power?
- How is power constructed and reinforced?
- How can we use our power positively in our influence with others? (Mannix McNamara, 2005b:4)
- What are the implications of reconceptualising power for empowerment practices?

Practitioners can be tempted to reject empowerment as they see a potential challenge to their own privileged position. The logical extension of encouraging people to question structures and processes is that they should be able to question the practitioner also. This can result in a mismatch with what is termed 'empowerment' but can actually in reality be assertiveness training, or feeling-good practices, with no attempt to address the internal locus of control or external conditions, both of which can be actively reproducing dominant practices of oppression. Assertiveness training is an important contributor to personal development. However, while it may be necessary for empowerment, it does not meet enough of the overall conceptual criteria for it to be described as an empowerment approach.

Focusing on this type of activity by health-promotion practitioners may be a means of operating within their own comfort zone. Real empowerment processes would enable the client to challenge both the practitioner and the external conditions of oppression. If the health-promotion agent makes no attempt to address the internal locus of control or the external conditions that hinder the client, then the practitioner themselves may be unwittingly (or otherwise) reproducing dominant practices of oppression.

If we accept Foucault's reconceptualisation of power as actively constituted in relationships, the belief that one person can actively empower another person becomes null and void. Power is not an 'object' that one person can give to another. One cannot 'empower' another person; it is not a benevolent gift that one person can bestow on another. One can only create the environment through which a person is facilitated to become aware of the implications of their sense of powerlessness (Mannix McNamara, 2004). Thus the focus in health promotion is not on building capacity with regard to *power over* another but rather is concerned with *power to* engage in action (Carey, 2000).

Empowerment is inextricably linked with Bandura's concept of self-efficacy. The feeling that one can effectively engage in action, and complete that action, is central to empowerment. Where empowerment is a consideration, self-efficacy with regard to capacity to complete the action is only one facet. The second and equally important consideration is fear of the consequences of engaging in a certain action. It is in this regard that Freire's raising of empowerment discourse into the realm of social justice becomes pertinent. Empowerment approaches are ontologically opposed to forms of oppression and exploitation (Mannix McNamara, 2005a). Health-promotion practitioners, engaging with clients and for whom empowerment is central to their process, must be cognisant of the social factors that may be actively hindering an individual's empowerment. They can provide support by addressing the psychological and social factors as much as is reasonably possible. However, it is imperative that practitioners do not give unrealistic expectations to their clients as this leaves an individual even more disenfranchised and further trapped in their disempowerment.

CLIENT OR PRACTITIONER EMPOWERMENT – OR BOTH?

The greatest dilemma facing practitioners with regard to empowerment is the expectation that they engage in processes that are empowering for their clients without any consideration as to whether they are feeling empowered themselves. It is questionable as to whether people are empowered to act in their organisations. Micro-politics regularly tempers how decisions are made. Lukes (1974) argues that systemic power can actually translate into institutional biases and people are not aware of how their relationships influence them either to use power or be the objects of its use. In other words, we regularly engage with other people and make decisions in a way that is influenced by the institutional biases that we have developed as a result of belonging to an organisation. It is incumbent on health-promotion professionals who actively promote empowerment for others to be critically aware of how they themselves understand power, how they use it and its implications for their practice.

In a study of how public-health nurses in Canada understood empowerment, Falk-Rafael (2001:4) found that nurses perceived the empowerment approaches they undertook with clients to be reciprocal in nature. They also asserted that 'they could only facilitate, not create empowerment in others'. From her study Falk-Rafael (2001:6) identifies empowerment as a process of consciousness raising, characterised by client centredness, reciprocity, mutuality, respect, enhancing dignity, being non-judgmental and creating a safe environment as critical to the development of a trusting relationship. Developing advocacy is also seen as an empowering strategy for clients and communities.

Empowerment is deeply complex but some general themes emerge consistently in any discourse related to it. Empowerment means different things to different people. Dialogue is an essential part of the process as it is through dialogue that the types of relationships and conditions needed are created for an empowering process and for outcomes to be possible. Empowerment is not static but rather is dynamic in nature and develops and changes over time. We argue that empowerment serves as an ideology of practice. It also serves as an act, a process and a psychological state (Menon, 2002). A key question for practitioners to ask themselves in critique of their practice is 'Am I creating the conditions for empowerment or am I manipulating so as to get the outcome I want?'.

SOCIAL CAPITAL

The concept of social capital has enjoyed varying popularity in recent decades. It has been argued that social capital is very important to the health, wealth and wellbeing of populations (Putnam, 1993). While some studies exist that link social capital to positive health status (Baum *et al.*, 2000), others such as Kunitz (2000) refute this, arguing that social capital can in fact be detrimental to health status.

Putnam (1995:67) defines social capital as 'features of social organisation such as networks, norms and social trust that facilitate coordination and cooperation for mutual benefit'. Trust is deemed an essential element of the successful functioning of these networks, as is reciprocity – the belief that the good turn done in support of an individual or organisation will be returned in kind. The return need not be immediate but it forms part of the networking process.

Baum and Ziersch (2003:320) describe the types of social capital to include *bonding social capital*, which they argue relates to the horizontal tight knits between individual or groups, and *bridging and linking* social capital, which can occur across communities or individuals. The sense of community, of social networks and of trust in relationships is central to social capital. One can often gauge a sense of the social capital by the level of volunteering that may occur within a community. Participation, which is a recurring theme in health promotion, is also an important element of social capital, as participation in community endeavours helps build social capital. Increasing links have been made between social capital and the level of health in communities (Wilkinson, 1996). Strong arguments have been made linking place and health, particularly that those less affluent in society have poorer health 'in part because the places where they live can be damaging to their health' (Baum and Palmer, 2002:353).

Social capital and health promotion are sometimes perceived as being incompatible, however, we argue that this is not the case. If we examine the principles of health promotion as identified by the World Health Organization (1986), empowerment of populations so that they take control of their health is commensurate with the development of social capital networks. Empowered communities can advocate for healthcare provision that is relevant to their needs. Tackling the determinants of health, including environment, poverty and social isolation, are priorities in communities focused on building social capital. Intersectoral partnerships with regard to improvement of health status are relevant to social capital, particularly in communities where networking occurs to reduce crime and improve amenities. Capacity building – both at individual and community levels – is prioritised in health promotion and in social capital approaches. The development of advocacy is central to health promotion and is a core strategy in social capital approaches. The five action areas outlined in Ottawa for health promotion can be argued to be action areas within social capital promotion also. The two agendas coincide tightly particularly in the areas of strengthening community action and the creation of supportive environments. The building of social capital and community development go hand in hand.

COMMUNITY DEVELOPMENT

Cox (1995) argues that community development can be understood as a process of developing social capital. Community development is the process of working with people to define their own goals and gather their resources in order to develop action plans to deal with the issues they have identified that need to be addressed as a community (Minkler, 1990). In keeping with the five action areas for health promotion as outlined in the Ottawa Charter (WHO, 1986) strengthening communities and encouraging capacity building so that these communities can effectively engage in advocacy is important. Processes of collaboration are central to community development in supporting those who are marginalised or experiencing social exclusion. The emphasis is on empowerment and capacity building for social change. In community development the task of building capacity is as important as the processes engaged in. Participation is also important as the community members themselves identify the areas of action and their resulting needs and action plans. This may be done in consultation with community development workers or by the community alone.

Tones and Green (2004:259) define a community as 'characterised by the existence of a network of relationships and a shared sense of identity, predicament or perhaps purpose'. They also differentiate between understanding community development as a *process* in which the momentum for change and development comes from within the community and community development as a *strategy* that may be necessary when a community is powerless and outside support and capacity building is necessary.

Perhaps the most famous protagonist of community development was the Brazilian educator Paulo Freire. Through his efforts to teach literacy to the communities he worked with, he came to some distinct conclusions that have subsequently served to influence health practitioners as well as educators (for whom his work was originally intended). Freire realised that in teaching, the place to begin was with the experiences of the individuals within the communities themselves. He perceived the potential of their untapped wisdom and set about building capacity among his students with regard to their critical thinking, and the literacy skills duly followed.

Empowerment of both the student and educator was an unexpected outcome of the process of building capacity and critical thinking. This translated into raised awareness with regard to the problems inherent within the communities. Those who had engaged in the process of raising their awareness also took on advocacy roles in order to improve conditions within their communities. The link between education and its potential for empowerment and liberation became central to Freire's work and has heavily influenced educators the world over.

Many community-development initiatives are influenced by the principles of empowerment and capacity building, which are central to the work of community development. Ireland has developed a strong tradition of community development in the past two decades in the area of health promotion. Programme development has played a central role in such endeavours. An example of an Irish community-development initiative is the Myross Community Development Network in Limerick.

The Myross Community Development Network defines as its aims 'To promote greater and more effective involvement of all the people of Myross in actions to meet their development needs.' The project is managed by people living and working in Myross. Some of the project's activities include supporting the set-up of new groups such as carers' groups and a residents' forum. They also include linking to other groups such as the Early School Leaving Project, promoting a positive image of the community through press releases, supporting the development of facilitation skills so as to effectively work in groups, evaluation of projects and the inclusion of those possibly marginalised such as people with disabilities, lone parents, prisoners, Travellers and asylum seekers. They also develop national networking with the Paul Partnership and the Equality Working Group among others. Careful needs assessment and strong attention to consultation processes are key to effective community development as the overall aim is to support communities in building their capacity from within so that they will continue to function effectively once the health promoter or facilitator has moved on.

5
Health Promotion, Lifestyle Issues and Work

Learning Outcomes:

On completion of this chapter the reader will be able to:

- understand the relationship between lifestyle, behaviour and health
- debate the relationship between health and work
- understand the dynamics of work–life balance
- discuss the role of organisational culture in workplace health
- discuss the role of workplace health-promotion initiatives.

INTRODUCTION

This chapter examines the link between individual lifestyle behaviour and health and the implications for health promotion. There is a particular emphasis on the workplace as a setting that can influence health and the promotion of health. The focus on work–life balance is explored. Workplace health-promotion initiatives are illuminated as are the principles and practice underpinning workplace health-promotion interventions. A discussion on organisational culture as impacting on employee health is also included.

LIFESTYLE AND HEALTH

The link between specific lifestyle behaviours and the risk factors associated with mortality are well documented in the literature. For example smoking, lack of exercise and obesity are identified as risk factors for coronary heart disease. Likewise, overweight and obesity are associated with a range of illness conditions, such as type 2 (non-insulin dependent) diabetes. It is not altogether surprising then that lifestyles are frequently the focus of health-promotion interventions. Indeed the focal point of health education traditionally has been on encouraging people to change their behaviour in the pursuit of healthier lifestyles at an individual level. The behaviours typically targeted in lifestyle campaigns include smoking, excess consumption of alcohol, substance misuse, diets high in fat and sugar and risky sexual behaviour.

LIFESTYLE APPROACH TO PROMOTING HEALTH

While there is a substantial body of evidence suggesting that much behaviour can be changed, there is doubt about how far health can be improved by targeting individual lifestyle behaviour or how sustainable such change is over time. Factors such as genetics and economic, social and cultural environment, which also contribute to ill health, are not directly amenable or responsive to lifestyle change. Therefore, targeting lifestyle behaviours alone will not result in significant health gain if the underlying social and economic factors are not addressed. Behaviour cannot be considered in isolation from the context in which it occurs. Take the example of Mary, a single unemployed parent with three children under the age of five, who eats a high-fat diet and smokes to help her cope with the stress of raising children on her own.

Within this example there are a number of behaviours that could be a focus for lifestyle-change approaches. It is obvious that a number of factors may contribute to her behaviours. If we look at her smoking in isolation from its context we may promote a smoking-cessation programme. However, on its own, such an approach may set her up for failure by not ensuring that alternative ways of coping are available to her. We need to consider whether Mary freely chooses to smoke or to eat an unhealthy diet. As health promoters we must be careful not to assume the role of expert by telling this person what to do and imposing our values on her, as this raises questions around whose needs and interests we are serving. We could educate Mary on the food pyramid and the ills of smoking so that she can make an informed choice. She may of course decide to continue smoking and we must then be prepared to support her in her choice. She may on the other hand be unable to make healthier choices because of lack of skills, or within the context of the social and economic conditions in which she lives. Should Mary decide not to take our advice have we failed as health promoters? This depends on how we see our role as health promoters and health promotion as an enterprise. If our focus is solely on persuading clients to adopt what we determine to be appropriate behaviour then we may feel we have indeed failed. Alternatively, if we see our role as educating, supporting and empowering clients to make informed choices, we have to accept and support them in their choice as well as the consequences of those choices.

The emphasis of successive Irish governments has been on encouraging individuals to modify their lifestyles. This is evident in Irish health strategies and media campaigns. Lifestyle approaches are very attractive to governments because they shift the responsibility away from government and onto the individual engaging in the health-damaging behaviour. By failing to assume responsibility for the factors that contribute to health, governments absolve themselves of the requirement to address the broader domains of influence on health status as outlined in Chapter 1.

This shifting of responsibility is often termed 'victim blaming', as individuals are considered 'responsible for the factors which disadvantage them but over which they have no control' (Naidoo and Wills, 2000:43). Whilst personal responsibility for health is important, the factors that are beyond the control of the individual must also be tackled. Some groups within society have consistently poorer health than others even if differences in lifestyle are taken into account (Nolan, 1990; Townsend *et al.*, 1988). As far back as 1974, LaLonde launched the idea that biology, lifestyle behaviours, social and physical environment and health-care organisations share equal importance as key contributors to health and should therefore receive the same consideration as determinants of illness or health. Authors such as Minkler (1999:121) advise that in health-promotion approaches a balance between personal and social responsibility is essential to facilitate individuals in making healthy choices appropriate to their needs. While the following sections will explore some key lifestyle behaviours, it must be emphasised that we are of the view that lifestyle approaches must be combined with efforts to address the structural factors that contribute to health.

PROMOTING PHYSICAL ACTIVITY

The value of physical activity to health and wellbeing has long been recognised. Galen, the Roman physicist who subscribed to a holistic view of health, acknowledged the centrality of exercise to his good health and longevity (Green, 1951 cited in Callaghan, 2004). Regular exercise is associated with a myriad of benefits to both physical and mental health. The health benefits of exercise for adults include reduced incidence of coronary heart disease, hypertension, stroke, non-insulin dependent diabetes mellitus, osteoporotic fractures, and some types of cancer (Bouchard *et al.*, 1994). Within Europe it is estimated that between five per cent and eight per cent of deaths are attributable to physical inactivity (WHO, 2002a).

The uptake of physical exercise can improve mental health, reduce anxiety, enhance mood and improve self-esteem, cognitive functioning and quality of life (Callaghan, 2004; Fox, 2000). Thirty minutes of moderate-intensity physical activity daily is recommended for health enhancement, while forty-five to sixty minutes of moderate physical activity is recommended to prevent excess weight gain in adults (National Taskforce on Obesity, 2005). Activity has benefits across the lifespan; however it is estimated that only forty per cent of the population engage in sufficient activity to achieve these benefits (Karch, 2000).

Shaping a Healthier Future (DoHC, 1994) identified exercise as one of six lifestyle factors to be targeted to reduce levels of premature mortality. This was built upon in the *National Health Promotion Strategy* (DoHC, 2000), which had as one of its strategic aims the achievement of increased participation in regular moderate physical activity. If these aims are to be achieved, then an understanding of the motivators and barriers to uptake of activity is necessary. Such an understanding will facilitate the development of a range of appropriate interventions to increase participation in physical activity. The *Allied Dunbar Fitness Survey* (Sports Council/HEA, 1992) identified the following barriers and motivators to participating in regular exercise:

Barriers	Motivators
Not being the sporty type	To get outdoors
Do not enjoy it	To improve or maintain health
Have not got the time	To feel in good shape
Need to rest and relax in spare time	To feel a sense of achievement

While knowledge of barriers and motivators is useful, it must be stressed that these factors may vary depending on gender, race, culture, socioeconomic group or stage on the life-cycle. Therefore specific barriers and motivators must be assessed for each individual or group when planning interventions. Families, peers, schools, workplaces and communities all have a major role to play in encouraging active lifestyles. Promotion of daily physical activity by teachers in schools can contribute to the development of lifelong habits. Family activities such as walking, cycling, swimming and pitch and putt provide opportunities for both family fun and parental role modelling. Becoming involved in local sports clubs and organisations in addition to enhancing activity has the added advantage of helping children to socialise with their peers rather than spend time involved in solitary activities such as computer games. Promoting physical activity at places of work facilitates those whose free time is limited. Community sports days, family fun days and the availability of local leisure facilities can also encourage physical activity.

In the mid-1990s, following the publication of the first national health strategy, *Shaping a Healthier Future* (DoHC, 1994), *Promoting Increased Physical Activity* (Physical Activity Group, 1997), a strategy for health boards, was launched. This document set the strategic direction for the work of health boards in the promotion of physical activity in their regions. *Promoting Increased Physical Activity* (PIPA) (Physical Activity Group, 1997) was significant from the perspective that it was the first noteworthy involvement of health boards in the promotion of physical activity. The review of the PIPA strategy (Physical Activity Group, 2001) highlights the ongoing need to promote the benefits of physical activity. The document also stresses the need to make physical activity more attractive, and to make it easier for people of all ages and abilities to be more active at home, at school, at work and in their local neighbourhood. Interestingly, it also lists some of the programmes implemented in this country to promote physical activity. These include:

- The Irish Heart Foundation's Lifestyle Challenge, which has been implemented in many health boards
- GP referral scheme: this involves a partnership arrangement between GPs and fitness and leisure centres whereby GPs assess and refer selected patients to fitness and leisure centres, where they undergo a fitness assessment and have a specialised exercise programme developed for them
- Slí na Sláinte: a network of walking routes to encourage people of all ages to walk
- Lifewise and Being Well: educational programmes
- Go for life Campaign: developed by Age and Opportunity.

Despite the increased involvement in the promotion of activity by the various health boards, the SLÁN surveys, conducted by the Centre for Health Promotion Studies (CHPS, 2003) reported that only fifty-one per cent of adult respondents engaged in some form of regular physical exercise – a slight reduction from the fifty-two per cent reported in 1998 (CHPS, 1999, 2003). Numbers of those who reported doing no exercise (CHPS, 2003) increased among men from twenty-one to thirty and women from twenty to twenty-five since the 1998 survey. Vigorous exercise rates are higher among school-going boys than girls. However, in the fifteen to seventeen age category, the gap doubles with a huge amount of girls reporting no activity at all. This is a worrying trend considering the benefits to health that can be obtained by engaging in regular exercise at all stages of the lifespan. In the CLAN survey (Hope *et al.*, 2004), which profiled the lifestyle behaviour of Irish college students, almost seventy per cent of students described themselves as fairly to very physically active, with males more physically active than females. Thirteen per cent of students took no regular exercise. However, it is encouraging to note that exercise levels are higher in this student college population than in a comparative group in the SLÁN survey (CHPS, 2003). The recent concerns about the growing levels of obesity in Irish children highlight the need to foster participation in exercise at a young age (National Taskforce on Obesity, 2005).

SMOKING

According to the European Health Report (WHO, 2002a:81), 125 million Europeans smoke and the annual death rate attributable to the consumption of tobacco products is estimated at 1.2 million (fourteen per cent of all deaths). Reducing the prevalence of cigarette smoking among adults is a key health-promotion target in countries where tobacco consumption is the major preventable cause of ill health (Graham and Derl, 1999). It is accepted that smoking is the largest single cause of preventable mortality and morbidity in Ireland (DoHC, 2000). At the end of 2001, eighty per cent of member states had bans or restrictions on smoking in public places and workplaces (WHO, 2002a). While plans to introduce a ban on smoking in the workplace in this country in 2004 were contentious and widely debated, the ban has now been in place for more than a year and has been a huge success. In fact it has been so successful that other countries such as the United Kingdom are considering following in our footsteps.

Legislation, however, is only one method of promoting health and various smoking-cessation programmes and initiatives are also common in targeting and assisting individuals and groups interested in giving up smoking. The stages of change model (Prochaska and DiClemente, 1984) is widely applied with varying levels of success. There has been a decline in the reported numbers of Irish people smoking in all demographic categories since 1998 (CHPS, 2003). In the CLAN survey (Hope *et al.*, 2004) twenty-seven per cent of all students were current smokers, lower than the number reported by a comparative group in the SLÁN survey (CHPS, 2003). The average number of cigarettes smoked was seven daily and males smoked more than females (Hope *et al.*, 2004). It is encouraging to note that one in four of previous smokers no longer smokes. However, reducing the prevalence of cigarrette smoking remains a huge challenge for health promoters.

ALCOHOL USE

Adults in this country have the highest reported levels of consumption and binge drinking per drinker in Europe (Ramstedt and Hope, 2005). Less than seven per cent of the Irish population under the age of fifty-five (CHPS, 2003) and only five per cent of the college student population are non-drinkers (Hope *et al.*, 2004). The numbers engaging in binge drinking rose from thirty-five per cent to forty-one per cent in men and from twelve per cent to sixteen per cent in women from 1999 to 2003 (CHPS, 2003).

In relation to the student population, males drink almost double the quantity that females drink (Hope *et al.*, 2004). Binge drinking at least once weekly is common among college students with sixty-one per cent of males and forty-four per cent of females drinking at least four pints of beer or a bottle of wine or equivalent in a single drinking session (Hope *et al.*, 2004). The rate of binge drinking among female students (sixty-six per cent) is almost double that of a comparison group in the general population (thirty-three per cent). Total alcohol consumption among college students is higher than that of a comparative group in the Irish drinking pattern survey (Ramstedt and Hope, 2005). Alcohol consumption has been linked to physical and mental health problems (CHPS, 2003), road accidents (McEvoy and Richardson, 2004) and suicide (Rehn *et al.*, 2001; Kendall, 1983). The high levels of alcohol consumption generally and among young people and college students specifically must be addressed.

ILLICIT DRUG USE

Illicit drug users come from all age, ethnic, occupational and socioeconomic groups despite popular misconceptions. Illicit drug use can result in physical and psychological dependence and can have devastating effects on individual users, their families, communities and society at large. Ireland has a relatively high rate (5.5 per cent) of opiate drug use (Kelly *et al.*, 2003). Cocaine and Ecstasy use has also increased in recent years (CHPS, 2003). Cannabis is the illegal drug most frequently used by college students (Hope *et al.*, 2004) with thirty-seven per cent of college students reporting that they had used cannabis in the previous twelve months and twenty per cent having used it in the previous month. Drug use among the student population (Hope *et al.*, 2004) is higher than that reported by the general population (National Advisory Committee on Drugs and Drugs and Alcohol Information Research Unit, 2003) in their national report on drug use in Ireland and Northern Ireland 2002–3. Health promoters must face the challenge of increased illegal drug misuse among the Irish population as drug problems reach everyone; users, families, friends, communities, workplaces and schools, and can lead to increased crime and healthcare costs.

DIET AND NUTRITION

The *North–South Ireland Food Consumption Survey* (Irish Universities Nutrition Alliance, 2001) indicates that thirty-nine per cent of Irish adults are overweight and eighteen per cent of adults are obese, with rates of overweight and obesity higher for males than females. In this respect Ireland is different to other countries where obesity rates are usually higher for women (Irish Universities Nutrition Alliance, 2001). The reported rates of overweight and obesity for both men and women have increased by three per cent for each grouping in the four-year period from 1998 to 2002, with fourteen per cent of men and twelve per cent of women now in the obese category (CHPS, 2003). The reported dietary intake of the population has also deteriorated with only thirty-four per cent of adults, compared to forty per cent previously, eating the recommended six or more servings of cereal, bread and potatoes per day, while there was an increase in those eating four or more portions of fruit or vegetables. While this indicates some improvement in terms of intake of fruit and vegetables, the issue of balanced dietary intake remains a concern. Conversely, consumption of fruit by school-going children has reduced by half.

There are numerous physical and psychological health risks associated with obesity including type 2 diabetes (non-insulin dependent), hypertension, coronary heart disease, musculo-skeletal problems, gout, osteoarthritis, low self-esteem, depression and eating disorders. As with other lifestyle behaviours a range of factors influences eating patterns including, genetic, psychological, sociocultural and environmental influences. Dietary requirements also change at different stages of life. Therefore effective health-promotion interventions must consider all factors in the design and implementation of healthy eating programmes.

SEXUAL HEALTH

The incidence of notified sexually transmitted infections (STIs) in Ireland has increased steadily over the past decade, with a rise of almost 178 per cent between the years of 1994 and 2003 (Murphy *et al.*, 2005). Recent national figures for STIs (2003) are higher for males (51.4 per cent) than females (44.1 per cent). The highest rates are reported among those aged twenty to twenty-nine years of age.

In relation to HIV (Human Immuno-deficiency Virus) and AIDS (Acquired Immune Deficiency Syndrome), Ireland has a low incidence when compared to other European countries. However, the frequency of diagnosis is rising. There was a ten per cent increase in the number of new cases of HIV (399) diagnosed in 2003 compared to 364 in 2002. The cumulative total of HIV cases at the end of December 2003 stood at 3,408. The figures for the full year of 2004 are not available at time of going to print. Of the 813 AIDS cases diagnosed in Ireland between 1983 and 2004 (O Donnell and Cronin, 2005), the majority were male (79.2 per cent). The increasing incidence of HIV, AIDS and STIs highlights the need for targeted health-promotion interventions. The HIV/AIDS campaigns of the 1980s and early 1990s were reasonably effective. Drug use (particularly sharing needles; blood transferred through the needle into another person's bloodstream), and safer sex (heterosexual and male-to-male sex) need to be targeted with effective health-promotion strategies to prevent the continued rise in the spread of HIV, AIDS and other STIs.

WORK–LIFE BALANCE – AN INTRODUCTION

Work–life balance is attained when an individual's right to a satisfied life inside and outside work is acknowledged and valued as the norm, to the mutual benefit of the individual, business and society (Jones, 2003). The emphasis on work–life balance has increased for a number of reasons. These include the growing number of part-time workers, the large number of employees who are working increasingly longer hours, the ageing workforce and the increase in mothers participating in paid employment. Recently there has been a greater understanding of the impact of work on health and the centrality of achieving work–life balance for health and wellbeing. Employers and employees may mistakenly associate work–life balance with parental responsibilities and may perceive work–life balance as a concept that applies only to working parents. However, a better balance between work and life is an issue for everyone, not just those with parental or caring responsibilities.

Work–life conflict

The negative impact of work–life conflict on workers' physical and mental wellbeing is increasingly being recognised by individuals, employers and governments nationally and internationally. Work–life conflict occurs when the cumulative demands of work and non-work life roles are incompatible in some respect so that participation in one role is made more difficult by participation in the other role (Duxbury and Higgins, 2001). A major constituent of work–life conflict is work-related stress. Working conditions such as heavy workloads, lack of participation in decision-making, health and safety hazards, job insecurity and tight deadlines are associated with work-related stress (Todd, 2004; Ryan and Quayle, 1999).

Elevated stress often leads to disruption in physiological and psychological health (Sarafino, 1998). A lack of balance between work and family life is a key factor in occupational stress. Occupational stress is a major health problem for both employees and organisations and can lead to burnout, illness, labour turnover, absenteeism, poor morale and reduced efficiency and performance (Edward and Burnard, 2003). Work-related stress is the biggest occupational health problem in the UK with stress-related absences costing an estimated £4 billion annually (Edward and Burnard, 2003; Gray, 2000).

The cost of work–life conflict

The cost of work–life conflict on individuals, employers, communities and governments is enormous. Work–life conflict impacts on job performance and rates of absenteeism, which are costly to both employers and governments. Those experiencing high levels of work–life conflict are likely to miss more work days per year, are less committed to the organisation, are less satisfied and are more likely to intend to leave their job (Duxbury and Higgins, 2001). Work–life conflict may affect the quality of personal relationships outside the workplace including relationships with children and spouses (Duxbury and Higgins, 2001). Children whose parents have more control over their work–life balance report less stress and are likely to be happier (Galinsky, 1999). Conversely, difficulties in managing this balance can negatively impact on parent–child relationships and the parent's responsiveness to the child, with implications for child health and wellbeing (Pocock, 2001). Work patterns, such as long hours and the strain placed on families in juggling their work and family responsibilities impact negatively on family relationships (CIPD, 2001 cited in HM Treasury and Department of Trade and Industry, 2003).

INCREASING WORK–LIFE BALANCE

The boundaries between paid work and life outside paid work are not as clear cut as we may like to perceive. It is not always feasible to keep work and home life separate. Children, for example, may become ill between 9 a.m. and 5 p.m. while parents are at work, which may result in a parent having to compromise with regard to their work commitments. Home and work life can become enmeshed. For example, we may bring work home to prepare for the next day, spend the evening sitting at the computer checking and replying to e-mails, never turn off the work mobile phone even when on family vacation. The boundary between work and home life is becoming more and more blurred. Indeed trends to increase the number of people working from home may serve to increase the blurring of such boundaries. Conversely the demands for more flexibility in order to be able to work from home, while sometimes argued as being more family-friendly, may also contribute to further complicating work–life boundaries. Fuimano (2005:24) asserts that 'people become enmeshed in their work so much that they treat it as if it's their life'.

Work–life balance does not mean an equal balance between work and other aspects of one's life. Trying to schedule an equal number of hours for each of the various personal activities in one's life is usually unrewarding and unrealistic. Life is and should be more fluid than that. Work–life balance is about people having a measure of control over when, where and how they work. It is also about how they combine their work with other aspects of their lives. A person's best individual work–life balance will vary over time and at different stages of life. It can vary for a myriad of reasons, for example, when an individual gets married, has children, starts a new career or nears retirement. Balance means different things to different people as each of us have different priorities and different lives. Therefore there is no perfect one-size-fits-all work–life balance.

This might best be illustrated if we consider one's life as having four quadrants. These quadrants comprise home (family and friends), work, community and self.

Figure 5.1 Life quadrants

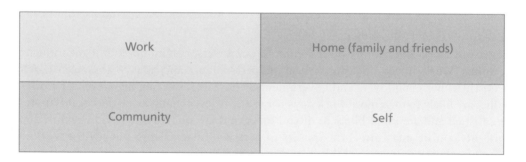

For some individuals, each quadrant may be equally balanced in the priority that it is given in one's life. The precedence given to each quadrant depends on each individual's priorities. Some may attempt to balance these equally and others may not, giving perhaps ninety per cent to work and ten per cent to family life with no time for self or community. Brown and Adebayo (2004:368) draw attention to the fact that for many 'the once-great divide between protected family time or leisure-time and work-time is rapidly decreasing as they slowly merge to the detriment of family life'.

HOW CAN WORK–LIFE BALANCE BE ACHIEVED?

The problem of balancing work with life must be addressed. We argue that increasing work–life balance must be addressed at a number of different levels. Clearly, as work forms an important life-context within the work–life balance domain, it is very appropriate that it should be addressed at a workplace level. Hodge (2000) suggests that 'Simple changes can make all the difference to all employees trying to balance their personal and working lives more successfully.' Employers for example may adopt policies and practices to assist their employees in reducing work–life conflict and supporting their different needs at different stages of their lives. Employees need to feel a sense of achievement and success in their jobs and in their activities outside of work to achieve balance. The work culture must be one where workers are valued, supported and respected by their employers. Trade unions through local advocacy and/or collective bargaining can promote strategies that support and enhance employees' work–life balance.

Some countries are more progressive than others in legislating for work–life balance. The Dutch government, for example, introduced the Adjustment of Hours Law (2000), which gives employees the right to request a decrease or increase in their normal working hours (the average is a thirty-six-hour week), which must be granted except in exceptional circumstances.

Similarly the British government introduced legislation which supports work–life balance by giving parents the right to request flexible working arrangements. At a policy level the Irish government is recently placing more emphasis on promoting family-friendly policies to employers. In its Programme for Prosperity and Fairness, for example, a key objective is the development of equality and family-friendly policies that support childcare and family life. Another Irish development is the annual Family-Friendly Workplace Day, introduced in 2001 to raise awareness of work–life balance issues within organisations. A Work–Life Balance Day replaced this in 2004 in recognition that all employees (not just those with children) need to balance work and other life demands. An Irish website dedicated to work–life balance has also been established (http://www.familyfriendly.ie/index.shtml).

So far we have concentrated on employer and government roles in addressing work–life balance. Individuals also have a role to play in enhancing their own work–life balance. Fuimano (2005:23) advocates for individuals:

> To balance your life, identify what doesn't work, eliminate those practices, then identify and add new behaviors. By eliminating stressors, you create the space you need to bring in the things you enjoy, and use your talents, skills, and strengths to create a happy and fulfilled life experience.
>
> (Fuimano, 2005:23)

Fuimano (2005:24), talking specifically about nurses' work–life balance, advises them to focus their attention on other areas of life to 'create a life that's energy sustaining and personally fulfilling', not just one of constant giving. This advice is equally applicable for a range of other occupations where the tradition of caring is a feature. Within caring roles, the potential for taking time for 'self care' has traditionally been undervalued and not always realised. Concentration on work–life balance is particularly important for those with caring responsibilities. Effectively managing time, reducing stress and setting aside time for *self* is central to achieving a balance between work and other areas of life.

WHAT ARE WORK–LIFE BALANCE POLICIES?

Work–life balance policies are policies that help workers to combine employment with family life, caring responsibilities and personal life outside the workplace while at the same time meeting employers' needs. These policies must reflect statutory entitlements like maternity and adoptive leave, *force majeure* and parental leave. While parental leave is available as a statuary right, take-up is not an option for many without income replacement. Outside the statutory entitlements, other programmes designed to help workers combine work and family life include job sharing, job splitting, flexi-time, term-time working, work sharing, sabbatical leave, part-time work and working annualised hours. Many employees may not be aware of such policies in their workplace. There is a danger that some organisations do not promote their family-friendly policies adequately.

Work–life balance arrangements have the potential to promote equality of opportunity among women and men by reducing interruption to careers. In the past, women often left paid employment to care for their children or others and in many instances this was not of their own choosing. Some returned after a number of years to a job very different to the one they originally trained for and in such cases their opportunities for career progression were reduced by virtue of this absence from the workforce. The Employment Discrimination Act 1998 prohibits discrimination. Within the spirit of this legislation, failure to consider access to work–life balance arrangements could possibly constitute discrimination on gender or family-status grounds.

THE VALUE OF PROMOTING WORK–LIFE BALANCE

While there are clear benefits to having work–life balance policies, relating to such issues as absenteeism, recruitment and retention and productivity, that impact on both individuals and organisations, Jones (2003:3) advises that work–life balance is 'a much bigger and further reaching issue than most organisations and individuals may yet have realised'. Jones (2003:3) argues that the smartest and most forward-looking organisations will see that by putting work–life balance at the heart of their cultures and strategic plans they will be not only satisfying employees and creating more equitable working conditions but also increasing their productivity and responding competitively to significant changes such as the growing 24/7 lifestyle.

In an Irish context there is an increasing economic need for those with parental and carer responsibilities to remain at or return to work. Some issues to be considered are the number of hours spent at work, the degree of flexibility available to employees and the autonomy that employees have in relation to hours worked. Some employees with parental or carer responsibilities may be in a position to work a full working week provided there is degree of flexibility relating to when and where they do their work. For some, reduced hours or work-sharing may enable them to successfully balance work and other commitments. A survey conducted by the European Foundation for the Improvement of Living and Working Conditions in 1998 found that both men and women would prefer to spend fewer hours at work. Women expressed a preference for a thirty-hour week while men would prefer a thirty-seven-hour week. They also found that more than eighty per cent of those working long hours (fifty hours and over) would prefer to work fewer hours (Thornthwaite, 2002). These competing demands need to be addressed.

HEALTH AND WORK

For a wide range of reasons, there has been an increasing interest in the relationship between work and health status nationally and internationally since at least the middle of the twentieth century (Ryan, 2003a). From a purely economic perspective, it should be noted that health- (or more precisely, illness-) related absence or unavailability for work means that there is a cost to be borne, which, depending on the particular country or its political system, must be underwritten by industry, an insurance system, or in welfare-type states such as Ireland, ultimately by the state (Cartwright and Cooper, 1997).

Work itself provides a very important social context for individuals and groups. The work status of individuals (being in paid work, in unpaid work or unemployed) not only helps define the social status and contribution of individuals, but is also related to issues of economic, social and health status. In Ireland 'out of work' income maintenance and support accounted for 0.85 per cent of Gross Domestic Product (GDP) in 2003 (OECD, 2005a). While this is perhaps a crude indicator when related to health and work, it is also interesting to note that of the overall unemployment statistics, 35.5 per cent of those unemployed were unemployed for longer than twelve months in 2003 (OECD, 2005a).

There is also some evidence that notable inequalities exist between social strata in terms of employment status, with those in manual forms of work being the most likely to feature in the ranks of the long-term unemployed (Jones, 1994). From a health perspective, it is noteworthy that long-term unemployment has been associated with identified risk factors which impact on health status and health-service utilisation, such as dietary factors, cigarette smoking and alcohol consumption (Department of Human Services, 1995).

Perhaps of broader concern is the fact that socioeconomic status has also been associated with risk of ill health or disease and is clearly associated with work status in its broadest sense. This in turn is not only a concern for individuals who are or are not in work, but also for their dependants. There is some evidence that suggests that socioeconomic issues in childhood or early in the life-cycle are associated with the possible development of chronic disorders such as chronic obstructive pulmonary disease in adulthood (Prescott et al., 1999).

Other conditions such as cardiac disorders have also been clearly linked with socioeconomic status (Iribarren et al., 1997; Lynch et al., 1997) and indeed socioeconomic status seems to be clearly associated with all forms of mortality (Kennedy et al., 1996). This argument seems to be equally true for physical and psychological disorders. For example, it is recognised that socioeconomic factors are important variables to be considered when undertaking risk assessment for depressive disorders (Jackson-Triche et al., 2000). This is borne out by the findings of at least one recent study with black women, where income was the socioeconomic indicator most strongly associated with depression (Scarinci et al., 2002). Supporting this argument is the fact that there is at least some indication that low socioeconomic status in childhood is related to a higher risk of major depression in adult life and that social inequalities in depression are likely to originate early in life also (Gilman et al., 2002).

While there seems to be an incontrovertible relationship between socioeconomic status, morbidity and mortality (WHO, 2001a), the direct nature of any causal relationship is open to debate. Because of this association, it would seem reasonable to be concerned with both employment status and indeed any association between worker health, the health status of those who are unemployed and economic performance, both at an individual and a societal level.

When we look at the issue of health and the employment situation, we can also see that health status has at least the potential to impact in a number of domains in one's work life as well as having broader concerns in terms of work. These areas would include such factors as availability for employment, retention, attrition, turnover and wastage, workplace performance, absence, sickness, productivity, employee and industrial relations and indeed attendant social costs such as welfare and insurance costs (Ryan, 2003a).

Examination of the literature on the relationship between work and health status reveals a number of important issues around work in its relation to both health and wellbeing. While there is long-standing and established evidence of the relationship between work and health, much of the research evidence has concentrated on distinguishing between the physical and mental health impacts of work or related to work environments. From the 1980s onwards, it has been established that a range of work-related variables impacts on health and wellbeing.

For example Rodin and Salovey (1989) report a number of factors that must be considered in relation to worker health. These include physical, chemical and biological hazards; physical demands; job security; psychosocial demands; control and decision latitude and social support. While these include environmental factors and contractual issues, demands and supports that can clearly impact on physical or mental health, other factors have been identified that impact on psychological wellbeing alone. These factors, identified by Warr (1987) and Waar (1990) include an individual's opportunity for control, opportunity for skill use, externally generated goals, task variety and clarity. Warr (1994) subsequently expanded this list to include availability of money, physical security, opportunity for personal contact and having a valued social position.

While there are some distinctions between these factors, there is also some apparent commonality. In effect these factors can be categorised as either external or internal to the individual and may impact on health status. This distinction is useful in that it broadens the discourse on health status outside just the individual and clearly includes the workplace environment. While much research has been undertaken to identify issues in the workplace that are related to health, it is also true to say that many of the indicators or risk factors are related to issues of ill health, disease or illness rather than health and in that regard, it should not be automatically assumed that the work environment has only deleterious effects on individuals.

There is an increasing realisation that workplaces can be healthy and health-promoting as well as having potentially negative impacts on employees. Work helps to provide individuals with a sense of identity, role and esteem among other things. Clearly 'positive' work environments have the potential to contribute to wellbeing and this has long been recognised. For example, there is some evidence since at least the 1980s that there is a positive correlation between high levels of support from supervisors and low levels of staff distress. This is supported by Stone *et al.* (1984) who found that supportive environments contribute to wellbeing. In their study they report that work settings where staff are supported by co-workers tend to make demanding tasks less threatening for individual workers.

Moos and Schaefer (1987) argue that there are two major advantages to these types of supportive and empowering work environments. In the first instance, workers who perceive their work setting as supportive and innovative demonstrate a greater sense of personal accomplishment, and secondly, workers with a high sense of job autonomy experience less emotional exhaustion and alienation. These 'psychosocial' consequences are in themselves evidence of an evolving trend towards greater acceptance of the significance of psychological factors in health and in economic performance in the workplace. As argued already, the traditional focus of work-related issues and health has tended to be disease- or disorder-focused and has concentrated on issues that are induced or influenced by the physical environment and external circumstances and conditions.

While traditions die hard, it should be remembered that more recent evidence supports the trend of taking greater account of a wider range of issues, based on the fact that psychosocial issues are estimated to be reported at least as frequently as physical hazards in work environments (WHO, 1994). It therefore seems wise that a holistic understanding of work-related health should be the norm and should ideally consider both subjective and objective elements of work life. This suggestion is also borne out in the findings of recent research on stress in the workplace among the Garda Síochána in Ireland (Taylor *et al.*, 1998b; Ryan, 2003a). The results strongly suggest that organisations and how they operate contribute to the overall wellbeing of employees as much as employees contribute to the organisations. Therefore in recognition of this reciprocal relationship, organisations must respond to employee needs in terms of organisational structure, design and culture; all of which contribute to the organisational milieu.

ORGANISATIONAL STRUCTURE, DESIGN AND CULTURE

We have argued that work forms an important element of life and a particular context. It should also be remembered that when individuals are in paid employment, most work within organisations, and we have also already alluded to the fact that there is an important interaction between personal wellbeing, health status and the role of the organisation. McNamara (2005) defines organisations as comprising 'a group of people intentionally organised to accomplish an overall common goal or set of goals'.

This definition draws heavily on the dual concepts of *intentionality* and *commonality of purpose*. This is important insofar as it suggests sharing and likewise that an organisation is a constructed entity rather than necessarily a natural phenomenon. Perhaps because organisations are contrived, they are normally reliant on some form of structure or design in order to ensure functioning. It is important to realise that organisational structures will vary between organisations depending on their function, but in all cases, the structures and design of organisations are likely to either facilitate or hinder the organisation's achieving the common goals already referred to (Chmiel, 1998).

Within the context of work, organisations normally have a hierarchical structure with clear divisions between 'manager' and subordinate roles. This classic structural divide can vary within organisations and the levels of complexity or layers of bureaucracy will differ on the basis of the size of the organisation and its function. Bureaucratic arrangements can either hinder or facilitate efficient functioning within organisations. Clear demarcation of functioning and levels of responsibility and accountability can help organisations to attain goals, while lack of clarity and/or appropriate levels of control within bureaucratic structures can lead to frustration and be associated with lower performance. The level and functioning of bureaucratic arrangements will, of course, impinge on the work environment, at least at a psychosocial level. In that regard, it is interesting, from a health-promotion perspective, to note that La Ferla (1993) proposes that there is ample evidence that the nature of the environments within which work-related activities take place strongly influences not only the quality of working life, work performance and safety but also general health.

The environment, of course, refers not only to the physical environment. While much of the research and literature on work environments has tended to concentrate on the physical environment, Cox and Ferguson (1994) argue that limiting the focus to the physical environment is erroneous. It seems reasonable to suggest that the totality of the environment needs to be considered if the causes, effects or dynamics of the work environment–health dyad are to be comprehensively understood.

For example, it should be remembered that organisations are dynamic entities that are characterised by political activity in its broadest sense. This type of activity is, in fact, fundamental to organisational life and is associated with power, authority and influence (Kumar and Ghadially, 1989). The type of political activity that characterises organisational life can be classified into three interrelated categories: methods of gaining power, strategies for impressing superiors and career advancement strategies (Dubrin, 1978).

The overall relationship between the work environment and health status is perhaps best understood as resulting from a complex interaction between physical, psychosocial and organisational factors and processes interlinked with the vital component of individual psychophysiology such as those referred to previously (Cox and Ferguson, 1994). This suggests that the ethos or culture of the organisation is at least as important as other aspects of the work environment. The politics within organisations is closely linked to the organisational culture. While the concept of organisational culture is difficult to pin down or quantify, Cooper *et al.* (1988) point out that where there is something wrong within an organisation, all involved know that 'something is amiss'. However a number of definitions are suggested. One definition suggests that culture is:

> a pattern of basic assumptions invented, discovered or developed by a given group as it learns to cope with its problems of external adaptation and internal integration that has worked well enough to be considered valid and therefore to be taught to new members as the correct way to perceive, think and feel in relation to those problems.
>
> (Schein, 1987:9)

Culture may refer to the deeply embedded traditions and assumptions that exert an influence on how a group functions. It can be both overt (written identity, beliefs, values and policies) and covert (hidden) and has been described by Senior (1997:137) as 'the glue that holds the organisation together'.

Clearly, within these perspectives, organisational culture can be understood as a powerful contributor to socialisation, and indeed control, within organisations. In many ways, the culture of an organisation incorporates both the tangible and the intangible elements of its evolution, history, aspirations, existence and the norms to which it operates. The culture of an organisation may be evidenced in rites, artefacts, language, ceremonials, symbols, legends, stories and the physical setting within or associated with an organisation. The health promoter as a change agent must take into account group culture and norms when designing or facilitating workplace health-promotional activities. Attempting to enforce any change that threatens norms invites resistance. Therefore culture and norms must be recognised and perhaps maintained, or alternatively the group must be helped to see how they are blocking innovation (Schein, 1987).

In order to identify organisational culture, it might be useful to remember that culture has been variously described in terms of 'typologies' as well as 'levels'. Handy (1976) describes four common types of culture:

- Power-oriented culture: a culture where the focus is on maintaining power and controlling those in subordinate positions.
- Role-oriented culture: a culture that is built around defined positions, with the emphasis on legitimacy, loyalty, responsibility, rules, procedures and bureaucracy.

- Task-oriented culture: a culture where everything is appraised in terms of its contribution to organisational goals.
- People-oriented culture: a culture where the organisation exists to meet the needs of its members.

Schein (1985) on the other hand describes culture as existing at three different levels. At the *surface* level are a series of artefacts (visible but often unclear). The *middle layer* comprises held values (greater level of awareness) and at the *deepest layer* are the core assumptions (often indiscernible or taken for granted). A very common metaphor that is often used to describe organisational culture and that reflects Schein's three levels is that of an iceberg. This metaphor is useful in that it visually represents the three significant layers at which organisational culture operates. At the visible level (above the water), usually the smallest part, is the overt culture of the organisation. This is represented in the behaviour of people, the artefacts visually available, the buildings and the structures within which people operate.

At the water level are the norms, attitudes and values (sometimes visible, sometimes not). This can be represented in, for example, who sits where and with whom. Who parks where, how meetings are conducted, how communication happens and how decisions are made.

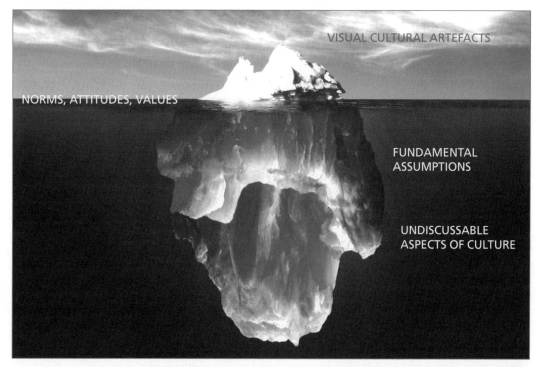

At the deepest level (invisible, but always the largest part of the iceberg) are the fundamental assumptions and meaning-making from which the organisation operates. Often at this level also are the undiscussable aspects of culture that have become embedded within the organisation. For example, how is power understood, who holds power, why is the organisation structured in the way that it is, who benefits, who decides and why? The analogy of the iceberg is useful in that icebergs float, sometimes crash into things and are difficult to control as they evolve a dynamic of their own. Venturing into the uncharted waters of any organisation's culture without taking time to critically reflect on its signifiers and on the implications of such exploration on future organisational development is potentially dangerous. For any change agent, it is important to test the culture and climate of the organisation before embarking on any change process.

Understanding the nature of culture and the elements that contribute to its development and maintenance make it possible to facilitate either its continuation or alteration. A positive culture can promote success while a negative culture, including one where there is dissonance between the 'official' or 'espoused' ethos of an organisation and the 'real culture' or 'culture in use' operating within it, can lead to failure to achieve goals and a dysfunctional organisation. Difficulties arise in an organisation when there is a difference between espoused goals and actual culture in that organisation and individuals within it may articulate one set of values but practice another. This may occur at a conscious or indeed a subconscious level. An example of this dissonance can be evident in healthcare where the espoused emphasis is on consumer involvement but the practice remains expert-led.

HEALTH PROMOTION IN THE WORKPLACE

Health promotion, as argued, is broader than a focus on individual health. Examples can be seen in the range of 'settings-based' approaches to health promotion, including healthy cities, health-promoting schools, hospitals and prisons. The Ottawa Charter (WHO, 1986) emphasises the importance of the settings approach to health promotion by its assertion that health is created and lived by people within the settings of their everyday life: where they learn, work, play and love.

The potential for health promotion in the workplace has gained increasing consideration since the fourth international health-promotion conference in Jakarta (WHO, 1997) where the settings approach to health promotion was emphasised as a central target for health-promotion activities. Tones and Green (2004) advise that a setting is not just a place or assembly. Settings-based health promotion involves a holistic consideration of the setting, its context and ethos. The settings approach builds health into the fabric of the system and ensures that the everyday activities of that system are committed to and take account of health (Naidoo and Wills, 2000). European support for health promotion in the workplace led to the formation of the European Network for Workplace Health Promotion, established by the European Commission in 1996.

It is not surprising that the workplace is identified as a key setting for health promotion considering that employees spend approximately sixty per cent of their waking hours at the work-site (Irish Heart Foundation, 2005). It also stands to reason that a healthy workforce and a supportive work environment will benefit both employers and employees. The relationship between work-related factors and the health of workers has been widely investigated (Gunnarsdottir and Bjornsdottir, 2003) and there is accumulating evidence that health-promotion programmes in the workplace can result in both economic benefits and health gain (Reid and Malone, 2003). American research suggests that employees who work for companies that have no workplace health-promotion or disease-prevention programme use the healthcare system more frequently than workers in companies that have such programmes (Whitmer, 1993). Workplace health-promotion programmes are also reported to decrease absenteeism, increase productivity, increase staff morale and decrease staff turnover (Orme, 2001).

Ireland, in line with other countries, has legislation relating to safety in the workplace. This legislation primarily deals with such matters as handling hazardous materials and lifting heavy loads, the focus of which is mainly on the prevention of accidents. Wynne (1993) points out that workplace health-promotion efforts in this country are prompted by legislation, accident rates and the perceived benefits of improved industrial relations. In that regard it can be argued that initiatives have tended to be reactive rather than proactive. Trade unions are mandated to work on behalf of their members for better, safer and healthier working conditions. At a legislative level, the Safety, Health and Welfare at Work Act (1989) obliges employers to identify and safeguard against *all* risks to health and safety. We argue that all of these agents have a role in collaboratively contributing to workplace health and supporting workplace health-promotion initiatives although some of these agents do not necessarily clearly identify with health-promotion activity as yet.

The increasing interest in employee health is reflected in the growing presence of occupational health departments in organisations. This, however, does not necessarily coincide with an increased emphasis on health promotion in the workplace. It has been suggested that health promotion is not considered to be of particular importance to occupational physicians (Cooper, 1997; Macdonald *et al.*, 2000). It could be argued that the main aim of many employers is prevention of sickness absence in working populations rather than a genuine concern for promoting the health and wellbeing of their employees. Indeed, employers' interest in health at work has traditionally focused on prevention rather than promotion. If we consider the case of influenza: if employees develop influenza this can result in both health effects and socio-economic and productivity consequences in terms of absenteeism. This has prompted employers to provide vaccinations to prevent influenza A and B viruses in employees such as healthcare workers to reduce work absences.

In an Irish study Reid and Malone (2003) asked participants (all the thirty-four human resource managers and a stratified random selection of 760 employees in the Irish Civil Service) to rate the overall importance of the occupational health unit and to prioritise eight proposed functions of the unit. The study demonstrates the differences of opinion that exist between human resource managers and employees as to the most appropriate functions of the occupational health unit. Human resource managers prioritised functions related to assessing fitness to work and pre-employment and promotional health assessment. In contrast employees considered preventative functions more important, such as medical screening, health education and medical surveillance. Interestingly the human resource management considered the department more important than employees, which suggests that occupational health units are more for the benefit of the organisation than the workers for whom they are ostensibly created.

It is noteworthy that employees in Reid and Malone's study (2003) would welcome a focus on health promotion and stress management in addition to health protection. Interestingly they emphasise stress *management* as opposed to prevention. While stress is one of the major difficulties in the workplace, self-help initiatives which are supported by employers can assist in reducing work-related stress (Beckwith and Munn-Giddings, 2003). While teaching stress-management skills is necessary and useful, stress management only deals with a problem once it has manifested itself. However the powerful stressors in the workplace must also be targeted for change (Murphy, 1998).

Much of workplace health promotion is centred on encouraging employees to partake in programmes designed to promote behavioural change. Such programmes include stress management, healthy eating, smoking cessation and increasing exercise. As argued elsewhere in this book, promoting healthy lifestyles is only one facet of health promotion and an individual's lifestyle behaviour should not be considered in isolation from the context in which it occurs. Kelleher (1998) suggests that interventions will only be effective if the environment is conducive to health and wellbeing. Promoting health at work, therefore, requires consideration of organisational and environmental factors, in addition to individual employees' lifestyle behaviours. Clearly, therefore, workplace health promotion should seek to improve health by empowering individuals to make healthier lifestyle choices. This may be achieved by a multifaceted approach, including the provision of a working environment that is health conducive, removing barriers to health in the workplace and improving the psychosocial work environment (Wynne, 1995).

IRISH WORKPLACE HEALTH PROMOTION

With cardiovascular disease one of the world's leading causes of death (Murray and Lopez, 1996) it is not surprising that cardiovascular health is central to many workplace health-promotion initiatives nationally and internationally. Their value is also well established. For example, positive results for diastolic blood pressure, total cholesterol and smoking for high-risk groups have been reported from some international studies such as a multi-component workplace health-promotion programme for cardiovascular risk factors in Switzerland (Prior et al., 2005). In the Irish context examples of workplace health-promotion programmes include Health at Work and Happy Heart at Work.

Health at work was a three-year lifestyle intervention programme. The programme, which comprised a survey, a year-long intervention programme and an evaluation, was undertaken in the health sector, at an academic institution and in industry (Fleming et al., 1997; Hope et al., 1998; Hope and Kelleher, 1995). The Happy Heart at Work (HHAW) programme was developed by the Irish Heart Foundation in the early nineties and comprises four elements: healthy eating, tobacco use, exercise in the workplace and stress. The Irish Heart Foundation supports the implementation of the programme and sets out a clear action plan which can be implemented in the workplace with the aim of developing positive attitudes and behaviour towards eating, tobacco, exercise and stress. An evaluation of Happy Heart at Work revealed that companies with in excess of 200 employees in the main took up the programme. Only 8.4 per cent of participating companies employ less than fifty people (Mc Mahon et al., 2001). The workplace was confirmed as an ideal setting to promote cardiovascular health and the programme fulfilled a previously unmet need.

One of the most influential national health-promotion initiatives at governmental level in Ireland is the ban on tobacco smoking in the workplace introduced in 2004. While it will take years to assess long-term improvements in health from the smoking ban, the occupational hazard that existed for smokers and non-smokers alike has now been eliminated for the health and safety of the Irish workforce. The introduction of the ban and the increased awareness of the health-damaging effects of smoking have inspired many employers to provide smoking cessation programmes, advice and support to employees who wish to give up smoking.

There are many issues to be considered when designing a health-promotion programme for the workplace. Any programme should be multifaceted and collaboratively designed in partnership with the employees. Areas to be considered when trying to introduce a settings approach to the workplace include, but are not limited to: work–life balance, communication, employee support, job control, decision making, health and safety, bullying, terms and conditions of employment, pay and other benefits, a culture where employees are valued and feel they are making a worthwhile contribution and where they are rewarded, team working, participation, policies and procedures.

6
Issues and Themes in Health-promotion Practice

Learning Outcomes:

On completion of this chapter the reader will be able to:
- understand the contribution of sociology and psychology to health promotion
- discuss the relationship between education and health promotion
- discuss the integration of health promotion in the practice of key professional groups
- debate the issues relating to health-promotion activity with specific populations
- define and discuss mental-health promotion.

INTRODUCTION

We have argued throughout this text that health promotion is as much an ethos as it is a practice area. Health promotion draws on theoretical perspectives from a range of disciplines and areas of academic interest. It is, or should be, an underpinning philosophy of practice in areas that impact on health status, both at an individual and population level. This chapter begins with an introduction to the influences of two key areas, namely sociology and psychology. A focus on health promotion within the practice areas of nursing and education follows. These provide useful examples of how health promotion is operationalised within key disciplines in health and education services. It also examines health promotion among specific populations that are characterised by social disadvantage or exclusion.

HEALTH PROMOTION AND THE INFLUENCE OF SOCIOLOGY

Sociology can be considered as a theoretical field or a disciplinary approach, but in either case the relationship between sociology and health promotion is a symbiotic one and therefore any text would be incomplete without exploring this relationship. Thorogood (2004) argues that sociology as a discipline is based on critical analysis and as such can contribute to health promotion by focusing on questions that go beyond simple definition. In other words, sociology can (and arguably should) engage in debate around why health promotion has evolved the way it has rather than merely trying to establish a static definition of health promotion itself. In this way, sociology can help health promotion to be reflective in terms of its role and development. While this means that sociology is distinct from health promotion, it is nonetheless a crucial contributor to the development and practice of health promotion.

Sociology as a discipline has two main foci. It is concerned with the structures of society as well as with the individual. At a *societal level*, it focuses on why things are the way they are within any society and explains them in terms of relationships, power and structure, among other things, but especially within the context of ideologies. At an *individual level*, sociology is concerned with why people behave the way they do within the context of their own environment, their family and community. Sociology is also concerned with the relationship between these two levels. The interaction between the micro- and macro-levels forms an important element of sociological discourse.

At a theoretical level, therefore, a major concern for sociology is the issue of social policy. It is in this regard that the interaction between sociology and health-promotion professionals or agents is most important. Health-promotion practitioners are concerned with social policy. Unlike sociology, whose main function is to critically analyse public policy, health-promotion agents have a specific remit in relation to such policy. While health-promotion agents are concerned with the development and implementation of health policies, they have a key role in the promotion of healthy public policies. Healthy public policies should not be confused with health policies, although clearly they are interconnected. Healthy policy refers to the concept of all public policies being 'proofed' for their impact on or contribution to health as a resource.

Sociology's concern with analysing and explaining the structures and relationships between groups within society is of pivotal importance to the functioning of health promotion. Health promotion recognises that there are inequities within social arrangements that may result in inequalities in health. Recognising imbalance is necessary in its own right, but it is more important to understand the causes of imbalance than merely to recognise them. Sociological perspectives on concepts such as 'power', 'bureaucracy' and 'social stratification' are therefore central to health-promotion debates. Health promotion acknowledges its 'political' role as being of primary importance and in that regard understanding the theoretical explanations of power, how it is established, maintained, or indeed changed, and to whose benefit or cost, become fundamental concerns for health-promotion professionals.

An understanding of the sociological ideologies and concepts is necessary for health-promoting professionals who are to act as catalysts for change. Engaging in sociological discourse requires health-promotion professionals to debate their own contribution to the maintenance or change of social orders within a given society as well as focus on the legitimate role of health promotion within a 'group' or 'individual' model of action. Such debates facilitate health promotion, as an entity in its own right, in examining its role within the power structures of society and at least focus the balance of its activity between broader 'sociopolitical action' and concentration on individual and community change. In that sense, it is only correct that sociology should critically analyse health promotion as a field of activity as well as inform its practice.

It can be argued that sociological critique contributed to the evolution of traditional health education into a broader health-promotion practice. Both, it has been argued, have the same intent (Whitehead, 2004), but the broader 'sociopolitical' and structural-level approach of health promotion means that the health-promotion agent has the ability to influence structural change. It can be argued that advocacy and empowerment approaches highlight the limitations of individual lifestyle approaches in that they fail to adequately address structural inequalities or tackle adequately the 'causes' of health imbalances.

PSYCHOLOGY AND HEALTH PROMOTION

As with sociology, no discussion of health promotion is complete without an acknowledgement of the contribution of psychology to health promotion. It has been argued that psychology has been the single biggest influence on both the theoretical underpinnings and practice of health education and promotion (Murphy and Bennett, 2004). This claim certainly seems true in relation to traditional health-education models, in that theories of communication, motivation, behaviour and change that have been proposed by psychology have been hugely influential in understanding human behaviour and change.

Before considering these contributions, it is worth reminding ourselves of the definition of health promotion. Health promotion is defined as:

> The process of enabling people to increase control over, and to improve their health. To reach a state of complete physical, mental and social well-being, an individual or group must be able to identify and to realize aspirations, to satisfy needs and to change or cope with the environment.
>
> (WHO, 1986)

This definition clearly suggests a facilitative role for health-promotion agents, with the key emphasis being on personal control over health. Psychology offers significant theoretical perspectives on issues such as 'locus of control'. Likewise issues such as self-esteem, perception, appraisal, cognitive and emotional development and functioning are key contributors to control and change. These theories and understandings have underpinned some of the key approaches to health promotion and education and have been referred to in Chapter 3. Interestingly all these theories refer to the key influences on change, whether or not they refer to behaviour change, attitudinal change or knowledge enhancement. In more recent times these perspectives have changed focus from individual learning to learning within and for social contexts. Theories such as social learning theory (Bandura, 1977) and the stages of change theory (Prochaska and DiClemente, 1984) have helped expand the explanations of human behaviour as well as the understanding of the stages through which individuals move in terms of making choices and change.

Another key area where psychology has added to health promotion is in the area of communication theory and practice. Since its inception health education has relied on the transmission of information between experts and recipients. Inherent to this approach has been the ability to communicate effectively. Psychology and communication theory have been central to all forms of health-promotion activity. Communication theory explains how messages are transmitted and understood. They inform approaches and best practice in health-promotion programmes in workplace settings and media campaigns at both individual and group levels. Therefore they are central to imparting health-promotion messages as well as understanding them.

HEALTH PROMOTION IN EDUCATION

Health promotion and health education are inextricably linked within Irish health-promotion practice. Areas of health-promotion activity in Ireland focus on community-based projects with capacity building as their central principle. We have argued that healthy public policy is a key element of health promotion. In that regard, education has been perceived nationally as a potential key medium for the support and implementation of health-promotion policies and healthy public policy.

We are now seeing a shift in focus in health-promotion initiatives from particular settings to a more comprehensive populations approach to health promotion. However, within this paradigm shift, there is still emphasis on particular settings such as schools. These remain key settings within which there is much scope for the development of positive health attitudes among young people via the curriculum and whole-school approaches to health promotion.

Traditionally, the educational approach to health promotion, or more specifically health education, as it has been called, centres on information dissemination. The presumption is that individuals who are given both knowledge and understanding of health issues will make informed decisions with regard to their future health. This model of health education seems to differ from health-education approaches in health settings in that it assumes that if individuals are given relevant information and simultaneously supported in exploring their values and attitudes with regard to a particular health issue then they will be able to adopt the relevant health behaviour. Therefore, the capacity of the young person to make free choices is an assumption underpinning health education.

Within this model also the health promoter is positioned as a facilitator of learning who provides the content necessary for attitude formulation and decision making in the health-education process. Internationally, the approach to health education and promotion in schools has varied, with some countries preferring a cross-curricular and whole-school approach to health promotion among young people in schools. Other countries such as Britain and Ireland have opted for a specific health curriculum to be implemented in schools. Health-education initiatives in Irish schools such as Relationships and Sexuality Education (RSE, 1995) and Social and Personal Health Education (SPHE, 1995) programmes draw heavily on the work of Kolb (1984) in which the experiential learning cycle is used as an effective strategy to encourage students to explore their values and attitudes with regard to their health literacy. Structured experiential learning initiates learning by designing an experience that the session begins with and in which the students participate. In SPHE the exercises are designed around a health topic. Engagement in the experience generates within the participants feelings, senses, and reactions to the exercise. The exercises can include activities such as role play, collage, reflection, brainstorming, self-reflection through life-line charts and so on.

Figure 6.1 Experiential learning cycle

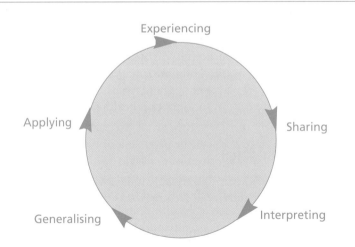

Source: Kolb, David, *Experiential Learning: Experience as the Source of Learning and Development*, © 1984, p. 42. Adapted with the permission of Pearson Education, Inc., Upper Saddle River, NJ.

Students then engage in sharing their experiences with each other in pairs or triads and then with the whole group. This facilitates the sharing of information and the comparing of notes, allowing the participants to test out their thinking in smaller groups before sharing with the larger group. It facilitates the release of any anxiety that may have built up during the exercise but also allows the student to recognise any potential significance from the work they have done (Graw, 1979). The tutor facilitates students in processing their insights and beginning to interpret them thus making sense of the situations experienced. By spending time on interpretation students are given the time to make sense of any significant themes and issues that may have emerged from their exercise. In generalising from the interpretation participants can begin to develop their understanding; they are then encouraged to apply new thinking and understandings to their relationships in the group and subsequently to generalise the learning to promote application beyond the group to everyday experiences.

Implicit in the use of an experiential learning cycle is the focus on attitudes, behaviours, knowledge and skills development specific to health promotion.

CURRICULUM PROVISION

The white paper on education, *Charting our Education Future* (Government of Ireland, 1995) and the subsequent Education Act (1998) advocate that education should be holistic in nature. The Act also identifies the need for an education system that caters for moral, spiritual, physical and social development for personal and family life, for community living and for leisure (Government of Ireland, 1995). These ideals, as set out in *Charting our Education Future* (Government of Ireland, 1995), mean that programmes such as RSE and SPHE should form a central component of the educational experience of children and adolescents. These programmes, therefore, should also be prioritised in education practice nationally, so that all students benefit from exposure to health education.

The introduction of RSE in schools at both primary and post-primary levels arose from the growing awareness among educators of the need to address the changing nature of society and the pressing needs that began to emerge as a result (Geary and Mannix McNamara, 2005). These included the fact that there was concern relating to perceived changes in lifestyle behaviours among young people, such as rate of substance use, sexual activity and suicide.

While RSE in-service provision for teachers and the curriculum itself was rolled out separately to SPHE, it was always the explicit intention that RSE would in fact be an integral component of SPHE (Government of Ireland, 1995). It is important to remember that the introduction of SPHE and RSE did not evolve in isolation. There was an established tradition of health-education programmes in many schools. SPHE and RSE actually followed pre-existing initiatives on the part of the Department of Education and Science and the Department of Health and Children to support the provision of health education in schools. Programmes such as the substance misuse programme Walk Tall (primary school resource) and On My Own Two Feet (secondary school resource) were already established in schools, as were the Stay Safe Programme in primary schools, and Bí Folláin (a primary school health-promotion programme from the North-Eastern Health Board).

While these and other programmes were already operational in many schools, they were taught on a voluntary basis. It was only with the introduction of SPHE and RSE that a coherent national curriculum focused on health education and promotion was introduced in Irish primary and post-primary schools. Currently SPHE is available to all primary school students and is offered at second level up to the junior certificate year. Curriculum and guidelines for senior cycle SPHE are currently under development by the National Council for Curriculum and Assessment and should be implemented in all secondary schools by 2007.

HEALTH-PROMOTING SCHOOLS INITIATIVE

The European Network of Health-Promoting Schools (ENHPS) was established in 1992. The focus of the network was the provision of school environments that were conducive to the promotion of health. The World Health Organization (1993) advocated the health-promoting school initiative and aims to achieve healthy lifestyles for school populations by developing supportive environments. There are currently over forty countries involved in the European network. For countries to become part of the ENHPS they must have a signed agreement of collaboration between ministers of health and education in their respective counties (Rasmussen and Rivett, 2000). In this way commitment to intersectoral partnership is evidenced. A management structure for the co-ordination of the project is necessary. In Ireland there is a national co-ordinator and a centre of co-ordination in Dublin.

While the concept of the health-promoting school is popular, the evidence of implementation levels is disappointing (Beattie, 1996). The implementation of a health-promoting curriculum is best served in the context of an environment that is health-promoting in nature. The development of a school health-promoting policy of which SPHE and RSE are an integral part would provide a coherent framework for the implementation of health promotion and education in schools.

THE HEALTH-PROMOTION ROLE OF THE NURSE

The health-promotion role of the nurse can be traced back to the emergence of the nursing profession in the nineteenth century. Florence Nightingale (1859) described her philosophy of nursing in terms of environmental factors that influence health and disease. Her stated goal of nursing was to 'put the client in the best condition for nature to act upon him' (Nightingale, 1859:75). Nightingale's focus on promoting individual and community health through a range of activities from personal care to political activism is consistent with contemporary conceptualisations of health promotion (Falk-Rafael, 1999). Other famous nursing theorists supporting a health-promotion role for the profession include Virginia Henderson. The value she places on health promotion is clearly evident in her definition of nursing, as follows:

> The unique function of the nurse is to assist the individual, sick or well, in the performance of those activities contributing to health or its recovery (or to a peaceful death) that he would perform unaided if he had the necessary strength, will or knowledge and to do so in such a way as to help him gain independence as rapidly as possible.
>
> (Henderson, 1991)

This definition includes states of 'illness or wellness'. Clearly implicit in the nurse's role is not only knowledge of health-promotion activities but also a health-promotion responsibility. Despite the strong emphasis on health promotion in the definitions outlined, nurses were traditionally more involved in the restoration of health and the alleviation of suffering than the promotion of positive health. This discrepancy between the values of nursing and its practice emphasises the requirement of nursing to move its primary focus from curative interventions and practice to both prevention of disease and empowerment of people to achieve their health potential. There are long-standing assertions in professional literature arguing that nursing has followed medicine in the move towards highly specialised technical care and a focus on curing diseases rather than preventing illness (Nagle *et al.*, 1999; Cloutier *et al.*, 1989). This has prompted claims that nurses' potential in preventive healthcare has been largely under-utilised (Robson *et al.*, 1989 cited in Nagle *et al.*, 1999). The same argument can be made in relation to health promotion.

The health strategy *Shaping a Healthier Future* (DoHC, 1994) proposed a health-promotion model of healthcare and the importance of the nursing profession in this model was highlighted. More recently *The National Health Promotion Strategy 2002–2005* (DoHC, 2000) advocated that the health service become a health-promoting environment. While the strategy document did not specify roles for particular professional groups, nurses, the largest of the professional groupings in the health service, are fundamental to the achievement of this goal.

Nurses have a key role to play in promoting change. Some authors, for example Hope *et al.* (1998:439), argue that this occurs 'at a personal level, as role model, as health promoter and as professional carer'. Within this suggestion, the clear implication is that the nurse may act as a role model or health-promotion agent at either an individual, family or community level. Nurses by virtue of their day-to-day contacts and therapeutic relationships with clients are ideally situated to promote health. An Bord Altranais in its *Code of Professional Conduct* (2000) emphasises the role of the therapeutic relationship in empowering clients to make life choices. Importantly, Peplau (1994) asserts that the changes clients need to undertake occur within the context of such specific helping relationships.

Nurses' understanding of health promotion

The complex nature of health promotion requires that nurses have a holistic view of health and be familiar with the myriad of health-promotion values, principles and approaches. It has been consistently suggested that nurses confuse health promotion with health education and use the terms interchangeably (Deasy, 2005; Whitehead, 2004; Maben and Macleod Clark, 1995). According to Maben and Macleod Clark (1995) clarity about the term 'health promotion' is a prerequisite to establishing the skills and knowledge required to practice it. Therefore, nurses can only effectively engage in health promotion if they are clear about what health promotion means. This suggests a need to increase nurses' awareness of contemporary understandings of health promotion and its relationship to health education.

Within the current educational preparation of nursing students, there are opportunities to develop the knowledge, skills and attitudes required to engage in health-promotion activities with individuals and communities. However, as this may not always have been the case, opportunities may need to be extended to all nurses to improve and update their knowledge of health promotion. Education must be combined with supportive organisational structures to allow nurses to apply their knowledge and skills in practice.

Nurses' attitude to health promotion

In an Irish study Deasy (2005) found that mental-health nurses have a positive attitude to health promotion and consider it an important part of their role. This is consistent with findings by Rowe and Macleod Clark (1999), who had earlier found that the majority (ninety-eight per cent) of registered general nurses in a Northern Ireland sample agreed that health promotion was an important part of the nurse's role. Duasco and Cheung (2002), in a review of qualitative studies exploring general nurses' health-promotion role in varied settings, including neuro-rehabilitation (Davis, 1995), general practice (Le Touze, 1996; Steptoe *et al.*, 1999) and community (Sourtzi *et al.*, 1996) conclude that nurses have a positive attitude to health promotion although their understanding of the concept is more centred on ill health than wellbeing. This may be related to the continued influence of the biomedical model of health.

Skinner (1995, cited in Whitehead, 2003) argues that most nursing models favour health-education approaches over health-promotion ones and relate more to individualistic biomedical than community-based approaches. Whitehead (2003) supports this view in his assertion that many nurses' health-promotion practices are governed by biomedically determined criteria. This is despite the evolution of a wide range of dedicated nursing models of care since the middle of the twentieth century. Nursing models normally articulate a perspective on the nature of health, the environment, nursing and personhood (Pearson *et al.*, 1996) and argue the distinctiveness of nursing practice.

The nursing process remains one of the most common ways of structuring care delivery within nursing. Reference to process suggests a dynamic relationship between caregiver and recipient and in the context of health promotion, information being shared and used for mutual benefit. This approach to care organisation has been criticised for being an inherently medical approach that requires a nurse to label a person and intervene with universal lifestyle-modification advice, often without acknowledging the uniqueness of the person or the meaning of the experience (Morgan and Marsh, 1998). Indeed, it is reductionist and in most instances has tended to be problem-focused rather than solution-focused or holistic.

This suggests that some of the models underpinning nursing practice as well as the means through which care is structured may actually hinder health promotion. Nurses must broaden the scope of their health-promotion practice to reflect the influence of sociopolitical, cultural and environmental factors as Nightingale did back in the 1800s.

Barriers and challenges to health promotion in nursing

While nurses acknowledge and value health promotion, it might be argued that the integration of a health-promotion ethos within their practice does not reflect the value espoused. They often hold priorities that are distant to their health-promotion function and fail to develop the role. This may be because of constraints in the clinical environment (Mitchinson, 1996; Deasy, 2005). A number of barriers to health promotion are identified in the literature related to general nursing. Lack of both time and resources as well as the reaction of patients to unsolicited advice are reported as inhibiting factors in research studies relating to district nurses, community nurses, ward-based nurses and midwives (Furber, 2000; Cantrell, 1998; Littlewood and Parker, 1992; Wilson-Barnett and Latter, 1993).

Barriers to health promotion in mental-health nursing include lack of time, staff shortages, difficulty accessing information, the stigma associated with mental illness and lack of motivation (Deasy, 2005). Interestingly, while mental-health nurses identified barriers, they distinguished these from specific challenges to promoting health in their area of practice. These additional challenges include mental illness, institutionalisation and staff training and education (Deasy, 2005). These barriers and challenges must be addressed to enable nurses to develop their health-promotion role. It could also be argued that reported barriers such as lack of time and resources suggest that nurses consider health promotion additional to rather than implicit in their role.

While there are barriers to promoting health in nursing practice there are also many opportunities. Within healthcare settings, there are numerous possibilities for opportunistic health promotion and nurses must both recognise and utilise these. This could include brief interventions using the stages of change model (Prochaska and DiClemente, 1984) in areas such as diet, alcohol consumption, smoking cessation, sexual health and physical activity.

Within Ireland, nurses are currently being trained in some health-service executive areas in brief interventions. The advantage of such training is that the interventions, found to be effective for a range of lifestyle behaviours, would only take up a few minutes of the nurse's time. Nurses must also embrace multidisciplinary, multi-professional and multi-agency partnerships to achieve the broad vision of health promotion proposed by the Ottawa Charter (WHO, 1986).

Health promotion in nursing practice

Whitehead (2001) proposes that nurses are unable to conceptualise the differences between health promotion and health education as distinct processes and argues that what nurses refer to as health promotion would often be more appropriately called traditional health education. Similarly, Benson and Latter (1998) assert that nurses predominantly adopt the traditional approach to health promotion, where the nurse is the expert who provides the information and advice and the patient the receiver of information. While providing information and advice is important this paternalistic practice may disempower clients and may mitigate against participation, collaboration and client-centred approaches that are key to health promotion.

Health promotion in practice is often centred on provision of information, education around lifestyle behaviour, skills development and individual as opposed to community empowerment. While individual capacity building is important, it must be complemented by efforts to maximise community capacity. Nurses have a major role to play in influencing health policy and addressing the wider determinants of health. While individual nurses cannot be expected to operate at all levels in health promotion, their potential power as professional advocates is currently not being realised. Structures must be established to facilitate and encourage nurses to contribute to health policy formulation and in an Irish context it was assumed that the establishment of nursing and midwifery development units within the health management structures would contribute to this process (DoHC, 1998a).

Strategies must be put in place at an organisational level that empower nurses to enable them to advocate for their clients, and within that context, these nursing and midwifery planning and development units were the medium through which nurses would articulate professional issues within the health management structures. A nursing policy unit within the Department of Health and Children was also established in the 1990s to contribute to policy formulation at national level. However, the establishment of these structures, while welcome, may not be sufficient to empower nurses to act as professional advocates and/or broaden their health-promoting roles.

Incorporating the principles of health promotion into nursing practice

Empowerment is one of the key principles of health promotion. Nurses, in addition to empowering individuals, must also work towards empowering communities, which is seen as key to improving individual and population health status. As empowerment operates at both the environmental (physical, socioeconomic and cultural) and individual levels (Tones and Green, 2004), nurses as health promoters must be politically active in confronting adverse socioenvironmental conditions. While the nursing literature underlines the importance of sociopolitical activity to health-promotion interventions, this is not commonly applied in nursing practice (Whitehead, 2004).

It is suggested that nurses, the largest health professional group, with first-hand knowledge about people's concerns, are ideally suited for social action (Morgan and Marsh,

1998). Indeed, Hewinson (1995) cites a body of literature advocating that nurses should 'get political', increase their collective power, become more involved in policy formation and play a central role in the shaping of healthcare. Piper and Brown (1998) suggest that nurses could collectively influence social policy to address socioeconomic inequality by lobbying power holders through their unions and professional organisations. Despite the calls for nurses to become politicised there appears to be a paucity of research examining the political involvement of Irish nurses. A national study in the USA surveyed nurse administrators on the reasons they perceived a lack of political involvement by nurses (Williams, 1993). This study identified lack of preparation in political activism, apathy and not being aware of the importance of political involvement as the principle reasons.

Advocacy is also central to both health promotion and nursing and can be seen as a unifying theme between both disciplines. Traditionally a core ethic of the health worker is to be the protector and advocate of the patient (Carlisle, 2000). Authors such as Woodrow (1997) suggest that nursing heritage has militated against advocacy as submissiveness to employers and subservience to doctors colonised the culture of nursing. The Department of Health and Children (2003b) emphasises the reciprocal nature of the empowerment of various groups; for example it is suggested that empowered nurses empower patients, while empowered managers empower nurses. Hewitt (2002), in a review of the arguments debating the role of the nurse advocate, concludes that nurses need to be empowered first, if they are to empower their patients.

Irish research exploring nurses' and midwives' understanding and experience of

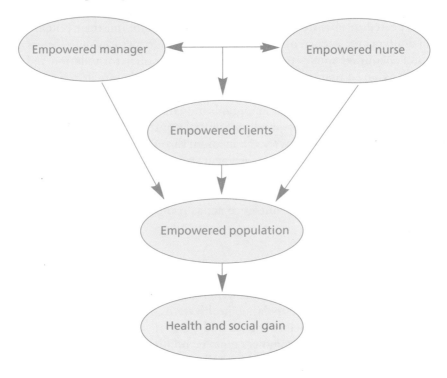

Figure 6.2 Empowered employees in healthcare

empowerment (DoHC, 2003b) suggests that the nurses in this study perceived themselves to be moderately empowered. The results indicate that education, knowledge, skills and self-confidence enable empowerment. Conversely, lack of education, lack of support (from management) and lack of recognition (from management and other professionals) inhibit empowerment (DoHC, 2003b). A key challenge identified in the study is 'enhancing the organisational culture to enable empowerment to become a positive element of health care in Ireland' (DoHC, 2003b:12). Therefore strategies need to be in place supporting nurses' empowerment before they are in a position to facilitate empowerment in others. Mental-health or intellectual-disability nurses, for example, specifically need to be empowered to advocate for those with mental illness or intellectual disability who are unable to assert their rights and whose families or friends may not be in a position to act on their behalf.

The importance of participation was brought to the fore by the World Health Organization's (1978) claim that people have the right and duty to participate individually and collectively in the planning and implementation of their healthcare. Maville and Huerta (2002:309) emphasise that whilst nurses are taught to include the client in formulating a plan of care, the client's input is seldom encouraged. They argue that nurses rely primarily on a professional-control model where professional expertise is dominant and clients are passive recipients of care. Clients are educated and it is assumed that knowledge will lead to behaviour change. Merely providing the required health information does not necessarily result in the modification of the patients' health-related behaviour (Whitehead, 2001).

Anthony and Crawford (2000), in a study investigating mental-health nurses' perceptions of user involvement in care planning, report that while mental-health nurses value the concept, many factors conspire to inhibit user involvement in healthcare planning. These include the perceptions of both clients and service users as well as their personal characteristics and beliefs, conflicting roles and responsibilities and organisational constraints. The failure of nurses to involve patients in any planned change may result in lack of ownership of the plan and ineffectiveness in bringing about change. Therefore, nurses must learn to pay attention to the needs and wishes of patients in order to promote their participation in their own health processes (Anthony et al., 1996, cited in Svedberg et al., 2003). Authors such as Sines (1994) highlight the complexity of the task involved in moving from a professional-led service to one based on the true sharing of power, such as in a consumer-based model. However, for health promotion to become embedded in everyday nursing practice, mutual decision making through genuine power sharing and acknowledging and respecting the patient's right to choice is fundamental.

Nurses as role models of healthy living

Yuro-Petro and Scanelli (1992) assert that healthy healthcare professionals inspire healthy attitudes among health-service consumers. This suggests that for nurses to be effective health promoters they must be role models of healthy living. Many nurses believe they should act as role models for their patients (Charlton et al., 1997; Rowe and Macleod Clark, 1999, 2000; Deasy, 2005). However, there is debate as to whether nurses can act as genuine role models for positive health behaviours, unless they model the behaviours they espouse (Soeken et al., 1989; Underwood, 1998; Deasy, 2005).

It has been suggested that role modelling healthy lifestyle practices can make nurses potentially more effective in their health-promotion interventions (Underwood, 1998). However, Rush et al. (2005:181) suggest that nurses who share their personal challenges and strategies for change with patients 'can be powerful in effecting behaviour change'.

Conversely nurses who continue to engage in unhealthy lifestyle behaviours such as smoking may experience cognitive dissonance in relation to being a health professional and a smoker (Festinger, 1957).

Nurses who smoke may have difficulty discussing smoking concerns with clients (Canadian Nurses Association, 1998; Rowe and Macleod Clarke, 1999). This raises questions around the appropriateness of nurses who engage in health-damaging behaviours asking others to engage in healthy lifestyles. Bandura's social learning theory (Bandura, 1977) suggests that one of the key means through which people learn behaviour is by observing a model. The dichotomy between the professional's engaging in unhealthy behaviour and making suggestions for client lifestyle change potentially creates a moral and ethical dilemma for nurses with health-promotion responsibilities.

However, research suggests that nurses who engage in unhealthy lifestyle behaviours do not necessarily feel that they cannot assist clients in changing their behaviour (Rush *et al.*, 2005; Deasy, 2005; Macleod Clarke *et al.*, 1990; Sanders *et al.*, 1986). Participants in Deasy's (2005) study argued that they could promote health despite being imperfect examples of what they were promoting. The image of nurses and patients struggling together to achieve health-promotion goals supports what Rush *et al.*, (2005:174) describe as 'humanising the role model of health promotion'. The participants argued that their honesty around their admission that they too have difficulties in changing their behaviour reduced the power differentials and actually enhanced the relationship, which was seen as key to health promotion (Deasy, 2005). It could also be argued that the participant's desire for egalitarian relationships with clients is not possible because of the contractual nature of the relationship, which is based on necessity, not choice (Ronayne, 2001). According to Ramos (1992) even in the most balanced of nurse–client relationships the nurse remains in control by virtue of their specialist knowledge and skills.

MENTAL-HEALTH PROMOTION

This section will define and discuss the concepts of mental health and mental-health promotion. The aims of mental-health promotion and the various strategies employed to achieve those aims will be illuminated. The potential benefits of mental-health promotion and the responsibility for promoting mental health will be discussed.

What do we mean by the term mental health?

In Chapter 1 we referred to the difficulty of defining health. Similar difficulties occur in trying to define mental health. It is our opinion that breaking up the concept of health into various components, such as mental health, social health, spiritual health and physical health, is overly reductionist in its approach. We also believe that using such an approach creates artificial divisions between physical and mental health and is inconsistent with a holistic view of health, which is more appropriate and in keeping with the ethos of health promotion. The tendency to reductionism is rooted in the notions of Cartesian dualism and historically is only a relatively recent phenomenon.

Cartesian dualism can be traced to the work of René Descartes in the seventeenth century. Prior to that, health was viewed as a holistic concept. Hippocrates, the Greek physician and father of medicine, born around 400 BC, believed health to be a state in which equilibrium between the mind, body and environment was evident. Galen, the Roman physician and philosopher, born AD 129, had a similar philosophy. The French philosopher René Descartes, whose work has heavily influenced modern-day thinking, is generally credited with drawing a distinction between the mind and the body. This led to a separation between so-called 'mental' and 'physical' health which implies that physical health is not to be considered in relation to mental health.

If you ask any individual what comes to mind when they hear the words 'mental health' their response is most likely to refer to issues such as suicide, depression or stress – issues associated more with mental illness than mental health. This is not altogether surprising as in recent years a shift in terminology – principally among service providers – has resulted in the term *mental health* replacing *mental illness*. Within an Irish context, psychiatric services, for example, are now referred to as mental-health services and registered psychiatric nurses are now more commonly called mental-health nurses. While the aim of this linguistic modification may arguably have been to reduce the stigma associated with mental illness, the change in terminology may have added to the confusion about the concept of mental health.

We stressed in Chapter 1 that health is more than the absence of disease. Likewise mental health is more than the absence of mental illness. Mental illness may be conceptually understood as the end point on a continuum of mental health within the context of a holistic understanding of health. However, for the purposes of conceptual and definitional analysis, it may be best to consider mental health and mental illness as separate entities. Mental health can be seen as a continuum ranging from optimum health to minimum health (including illness states) rather than an absolute state.

Mental health has been variously defined in the literature. For example, Fontaine (2003:45) suggests that mental health is a 'lifelong process and includes a sense of harmony and balance for the individual, family, friends and community'. The UK Health Education Authority in its *Mental Health Promotion: A Quality Framework* (1997) defines mental health as the emotional and spiritual resilience which enable us to enjoy life and to survive pain, suffering and disappointment. It is a positive sense of wellbeing and an underlying belief in our own and others' dignity and worth. It is a resource which we need for everyday life, which enables us to manage our lives successfully (Health Education Authority, 1997).

These definitions suggest a number of important dimensions. The idea of process in Fontaine's definition is interesting. This concept of process within a relationship between individuals, concerned persons and the wider community suggests a transactional understanding. Likewise, this understanding is also evident in the second definition in that it argues that one of the key dimensions against which mental health may be measured is the balance in all aspects of people's lives. How we feel about others and ourselves and how we cope with everyday demands is central to mental health. Mental health, therefore, is – or should be – of interest to us all, not just to those who have mental illness.

In Chapter 1 we identified a number of factors that impact on our experience of health. As mental health is an integral dimension of overall health, these factors obviously impact on mental wellbeing also. Within the context of a transactional understanding of mental health, there are a number of factors which, we would suggest, positively influence mental health. These include social competence, positive self-esteem, good physical health, appropriate coping and life skills, the ability to deal with change, being involved in supportive relationships, adequate resources and having access to support services. Factors which can negatively impact on mental health include poor interpersonal relationships, unmet needs, low self-esteem, inadequate or inappropriate social and coping skills, the inability to communicate or express feelings, having a physical illness or disability, social isolation, poverty and unemployment.

Defining mental-health promotion
Mental-health promotion in its broadest sense refers to any action taken to enhance the mental health of individuals, groups or communities. Hodgson stresses the centrality of capacity building to mental-health promotion in his definition:

> Mental health promotion can de defined as the enhancement of the capacity of individuals, families, groups or communities to strengthen or support positive emotional cognitive and related experiences.

> (Hodgson 1996:2)

This definition is interesting from an overall health-promotion perspective. Clearly the idea of capacity building at an individual, group and social level is central to this definition. If we accept that mental health is a continuum ranging from optimum health to minimum health, it follows that efforts to promote mental health must be concerned with two key 'capacity' issues. On the one hand, mental-health promotion must be concerned with 'supportive actions' such as augmenting the factors that contribute to optimal mental health and simultaneously reducing the factors that contribute to minimal mental-health states. In addition mental-health promotion is concerned with the factors which inhibit individuals' achievement of optimal mental-health status. These approaches will also clearly empower individuals.

The aims of mental-health promotion
Taylor (1998a) describes the aim of mental-health-promotion approaches as three-fold: to enhance protective factors, to decrease risk factors for poor mental health and to reduce inequities among populations. This tripartite model is consistent with our suggestion of capacity building, support and empowerment.

Activities to enhance protective factors focus on strengthening the ability of individuals, families or communities to cope with events that happen in their everyday lives. Examples include facilitating self-help networks; increasing life skills, social skills and coping skills; enhancing self-esteem and self-acceptance and strengthening social support. Activities which aim to decrease risk factors include efforts to reduce anxiety, depression, stress, suicide, helplessness, abuse, substance misuse, violence and social isolation. Activities to reduce inequities among populations focus on issues such as lack of access to services because of poverty or geographical location; discrimination on grounds of gender, sexuality, race or disability; community insecurity; poor quality housing or unemployment (Taylor, 1998a).

Strategies for promoting mental health
Mental-health-promotion strategies are diverse and can range from developing the personal skills of individuals to reducing structural barriers to health. A summary of mental-health-promotion strategies (approaches) is provided below:

Approaches to mental-health promotion
- capacity building of individuals and communities
- advocacy
- increasing community understanding and awareness of mental health and mental illness
- reducing health inequalities and other major structural barriers to health

- contributing to health policy and healthy public policy
- targeting select population groups such as children, adolescents, third-level students, adults, older adults
- targeting at-risk groups, for example long-term carers, young males, those experiencing bereavement, Travellers and the homeless (to name just a few)
- reducing stigma and discrimination for those with ongoing mental-health problems
- ensuring that those with existing mental-health problems maximize their opportunity for full and lasting recovery
- researching to generate knowledge on which future programmes are based

Examples of national programmes currently operating to promote mental health include:

- Mental Health Matters and The National Public Speaking Project run by Mental Health Ireland which aim to increase awareness of mental health
- RSE and SPHE programmes in schools
- The Community Mothers Programme targeted at disadvantaged first- and second-time parents of children under two
- Parenting programmes
- Fás le Cheile (NWHB) a programme that promotes positive relationships between parents and young children
- The Mind Out programme: mental-health promotion module for senior-cycle students
- Mental health days
- Cool School anti bullying programme (NWHB)

The potential benefits of mental-health promotion
The potential benefits of mental-health promotion are extensive. Mental-health promotion can strengthen the capacity of individuals and communities. It can lead to improved physical health and wellbeing. It can help to reduce the structural barriers to mental health. Mental-health promotion can help to prevent or reduce the risk of some mental-health problems. For example reducing stress can help prevent depression in some individuals. For those individuals with mental-health problems it can assist with recovery and enhance quality of life through supportive and empowering interventions. By creating awareness of mental health and the continuum model, it can help to reduce the stigma and discrimination so often experienced by those with mental illness. In that way it is also presumed that it will potentially lead to early recognition of health problems and early intervention. Indeed this was possibly the early focus of mental-health-promotion activity; namely awareness raising, illness recognition, prevention and early intervention.

Improving the health of workers has the potential to increase productivity and to reduce days lost through illness. Promoting the mental health of children may increase their resilience and in turn reduce their potential for mental-health problems in adulthood.

This list is by no means complete but provides an indication of the possibilities for health and social gain that can be achieved through the promotion of mental health.

Responsibility for mental-health promotion
Historically mental and physical health promotion developed as separate entities, largely because of the philosophical underpinnings of the medical model of care on which most western health services are based. As argued earlier, this model is reductionist and sees

domains of health as being separate, distinct and unrelated. In that model there is a dichotomy between the mind and the body and this reflected itself in tendencies in the health services to consider cognitive and emotional aspects of health as being unrelated to physical health.

However, in more recent times there is an increasing recognition and acceptance of the fact that physical and mental health are clearly interrelated and in fact interdependent for overall wellbeing. Physical wellbeing has a significant influence on mental health and mental health is imperative in the maintenance of good physical health and recovery from physical illness (Herrman, 2001). There is increasing evidence in the professional literature of this relationship. For example, studies indicate relationships between mental-health problems and poor physical health. Those with mental-health problems are at increased risk of mortality from cardiovascular disease and respiratory infection, and there is a greater prevalence of hepatitis C and diabetes among those with mental-health problems (Friedli and Dardis, 2002; Phelan *et al.*, 2001; Davidson *et al.*, 2001a; Davidson *et al.*, 2001b; Harris and Baraclough, 1998). Conversely, those with physical health disorders such as stroke, cancer and arthritis experience higher rates of mental illness. The reciprocal relationship between mental and physical health underlines the centrality to health promotion of a holistic view of individuals.

Despite a strong body of evidence identifying the reciprocal relationship between mental and physical health, it is interesting that this holistic understanding is not adequately reflected in either health-service provision arrangements or in health-promotion activity generally. The mental-health services in Ireland have been under ongoing restructuring since the publication of a key policy document titled *Psychiatric Services: Planning for the Future* in the mid-1980s (DoHC, 1984). Part of that restructuring involved the development of acute inpatient services attached to general hospitals and the development of community-based services.

However, no matter how welcome this development is, some of the main reasons for it were to normalise mental illness and reduce stigma associated with mental illness. While these aims are laudable, they are aimed at illness management and recovery, rather than health promotion and illness prevention. In an Irish context, the tendency has been that mental-health promotion has traditionally been undertaken mainly by health practitioners in tertiary mental-health services rather than health-promotion practiioners. This seems somewhat contradictory and incongruent, given that the focus of most mental-health services in Ireland as well as internationally is on the management of illness conditions. Therefore it can be argued that despite strong evidence, a health promotion–mental-health promotion dichotomy continues today.

In Ireland, while much mental-health promotion has been associated with tertiary mental-health services, it is also true to say that responsibility for mental-health promotion has historically been shared between the Department of Health and Children and voluntary and community groups such as women's groups, youth groups and mental-health organisations (Brennan, 2000). There are quite a number of voluntary agencies which are actively involved in promoting mental health. These include groups such as Mental Health Ireland, Schizophrenia Ireland, the Out and About Association, Aware, Grow and Bodywhys to name just a few. According to Brennan (2000) many of the organisations involved in mental-health promotion have a dual mandate: to improve psychiatric services and to promote positive mental health. This is clearly problematic from the perspective of being overly associated with health-service improvement and being part of a service primarily associated with an illness focus.

The separation of mental and physical health is inconsistent with a holistic view of health and of individuals, which is a fundamental assumption of health promotion. This fragmentation has not been unnoticed internationally. Indeed there have been calls for the activities of mental-health promotion to be mainstreamed with health promotion (Herrman, 2001; WHO, 2001b). Considering that mental health is integral to overall health it is our opinion that mental-health promotion should be an integral part of health promotion in general rather than a separate entity.

Many health professionals are engaged in mental-health promotion. These include, but are not limited to, psychiatric nurses, general practitioners, psychiatrists, psychologists, social workers and occupational therapists. Mental-health promotion is considered central to the role of the psychiatric nurse. The objective of psychiatric nursing according to An Bord Altranais (2005:27) is to 'facilitate the maximum development of the mental health of the individual who has psychiatric problems and to promote mental health'. In addition the mental-health nurse has a role in restoring and maintaining mental health and an educative role in the prevention of psychiatric illness.

Despite the emphasis on mental-health promotion, the focus of psychiatric and mental-health nursing practice, as in other branches of nursing, has traditionally concentrated on the care of the ill at the expense of health promotion and illness prevention (Ryan, 2003b). This is not surprising when you consider the influence of the binary medical model on the education and training of psychiatric nurses and indeed in all areas of health-service provision. In a recent qualitative study, Deasy (2005) found that while psychiatric nurses promoted the mental health of their clients, most were not involved in promoting the mental health of the wider community. Many perceived that they could have a greater role in creating awareness and reducing stigma.

While many professionals have a responsibility to promote mental health it is obvious that many of the factors that influence mental health are outside the remit of the health service. These can only be tackled through a co-ordinated multisectoral approach which focuses on whole populations, individuals at risk, vulnerable groups and those with existing mental-health problems. This requires resources and a partnership approach across a range of sectors, disciplines, agencies and departments. It also requires a shared vision and strategic planning.

Over the past decade both nationally and internationally there is increasing recognition that mental health is an integral part of health and therefore must be addressed to achieve improvements in overall health and wellbeing. Murray and Lopez (1996) estimate that depression will constitute one of the greatest health problems worldwide by 2020. Ireland has one of the fastest rising rates of suicide in the world. In 2001 448 people died by suicide in Ireland – one per cent of all deaths (National Suicide Review Group, 2001). Suicide was found to be the second biggest cause of death in the fifteen to twenty-four age group overall and almost eighty per cent of suicides were carried out by males (National Suicide Review Group, 2001). While the primary focus of health promotion and *inter alia* mental-health promotion should correctly be on capacity building, support and empowerment, this data suggests that another clear domain of activity relates to illness and mortality prevention. Health promotion has a role to play in preventing some types of mental illness and improving the quality of life for those with mental-health problems. Promoting mental health is also an important aspect of suicide prevention. This can be achieved through the types of activity (capacity building, support and empowerment) referred to earlier.

At international level, organisations such as the World Health Organization, the World Psychiatric Association and the World Federation for Mental Health are key players in strengthening the value placed on mental health. Nationally, while a mental-health promotion strategy is planned it has not yet been published. It is hoped that this strategy will provide a strategic, synchronised and targeted approach to mental-health promotion in Ireland in the coming years. Yet at the same time, while a dedicated emphasis on aspects of mental health may be welcome, as it can be argued that mental health was a forgotten or hidden aspect of health for too long, it is equally arguable that it would be more conceptually consistent were mental-health promotion to be situated within an overall health-promotion strategy. This is argued in the context of other strategy documents published over the past decade. Many of these have highlighted the need for promoting mental health. The health-promotion strategy *Making the Healthier Choice the Easier Choice* (DoHC, 1995:26) listed as one of its goals 'to promote mental health in cooperation with the voluntary mental health bodies and the health boards'.

It also identified the following actions needed to realise this goal:

- Providing programmes that develop mental and emotional health, self esteem, personal relationships and coping skills.
- Strengthening the individual's basic capacity to make healthy choices and to cope with stressful situations without recourse to behaviours which may damage health.
- Continuing support for an intervention study at reducing the prevalence and cost of suicide.

(DoHC, 1995:26)

While it is significant that action goals were included in this document they relate to health promotion at an individual level and make no reference to the health of the community or indeed to addressing the structural barriers to achieving mental health. Other strategies which followed, such as the *National Health Promotion Strategy* (DoHC, 2000), *The Health of Our Children* (DoHC, 2001d), the *Adolescent Health Strategy* (DoHC, 2001a) and *Quality and Fairness: A Health System for You* (DoHC, 2001b) have highlighted the need for enhancing and promoting mental health.

Regional strategies have also been developed, for example the North-Western Health Board's strategy for *Mental Health into the Millennium and Beyond* (2000). Mental-health promotion has also been recommended in recent reports, for example three of the ten recommendations arising from the CLAN survey (Hope *et al.*, 2004) specifically relate to promoting mental health. Recommendation number two (page 16) states:

Health promotion structures and frameworks should give priority to mental-health promotion and reducing alcohol related harm.

Recommendation number seven (page 16) states:

Colleges should be encouraged to develop and implement an action plan for mental-health promotion with emphasis on enhancing the protective factors including circle of friends as key contacts and reducing risk factors such as alcohol related harm.

Recommendation number nine (page 16) states:

College clubs and societies should seek opportunities to promote positive health with strategies to promote mental health and low risk drinking.

Quality and Fairness (DoHC, 2001b) recommended reorienting the health system towards primary-care provision. It is our opinion that this reorientation can provide scope for planned and opportunistic mental-health promotion through the day-to-day contacts between health professionals and individuals in their community. Through health education with clients and advocacy on behalf of their community, primary healthcare personnel can support individual needs and influence the policies and programmes that affect the mental health of the community.

The increasing recognition and value placed on mental health to achieve health gain is welcome. It is our opinion that this could be achieved more effectively if the bodies engaged in mental-health promotion and those promoting health generally worked collectively and collaboratively in an integrated manner, rather than separately, to promote health holistically.

ETHNICITY, CULTURE AND HEALTH PROMOTION

In our earlier discussion on the definition of health and health promotion, we argued that health is not an end in its own right, but rather a resource for living. We also argued that health promotion is not a discrete area of activity, but rather one that incorporates a wide variety of perspectives and is epitomised as an approach as opposed to a singular activity. In other words, it is an ethos incorporated within a range of disciplines and sectors at a variety of levels. It aims for an integrated, inter- or trans-sectoral approach that is holistic and focused on health as a resource for living. It addresses health and social inequalities so as to enable individuals and groups to live life to the optimum. It achieves these aims through such approaches as empowerment, individual and community support, political activity and policy-level intervention among others. These aims, objectives and areas of activity are important when we consider specific populations or discrete groups within society.

We can, of course, argue that considering discrete groups within an overall population is reductionist and conceptually at odds with holistic health-promotion principles. While this may be at least partly true, it is equally true to argue that inequalities should be targeted within the overall context of population health and therefore providing special attention to specific groups becomes legitimate.

Despite philosophical concerns and debates, we must remember that the overall purpose of promoting health is to enhance the opportunities of people to maximise their life experience and opportunities. In doing so, it must be considered that people live within broader societies and that in turn leads us to consider the notion of citizenship. Citizenship has traditionally been associated with nationality and a definite link to a particular country or nation state. Indeed within the debates relating to citizenship, at least two divergent perspectives emerge.

In the first instance, citizenship can be understood to be a status which someone has – normally based on their birth or allegiance to a state or nation. In this context, citizenship is understood to be a right (or a set of rights) that someone has conferred on them automatically by virtue of this membership of the community. Alternatively, citizenship can be seen as a status achieved by virtue of someone's contribution to or engagement with a community (Plant, 2003). Normally, though not exclusively, the community is synonymous with a political community or a state. Within a European context, the evolution of the European Economic Community through a variety of treaties to its current incarnation as the European Union has been testament to a changing notion of citizenship, with shared rights across national borders. Frequent reference is now made to EU citizens and non-EU citizens, and while this reference may be more correctly described as EU or non-EU state citizens, the term has come into popular usage and shared meaning. Indeed, in that context the case of ethnic groupings makes for interesting discussion in relation to social inclusion, cohesion and citizenship as either a right or an obligation. In either context, if we assume that health is a right, as stipulated by the Universal Declaration of Human Rights (United Nations, 1948), or a necessary prerequisite to contribute to society, then ethnic groups, refugees and asylum seekers are particular populations that provide interesting points of discourse.

Multiculturalism and health promotion

The social and political reality of the early twenty-first century means that population movement at an individual and group level is the accepted norm. Across Europe and elsewhere the issue of migration and the management of ethnic groups within society is an issue of considerable debate. Migration has become an increasing trend in western civilisations with globalisation and this in turn raises the importance of health and social-service agencies taking due cognisance of ethnicity and cultural diversity.

Ethnic and cultural concerns are sometimes confused with situations of forced migration. Indeed it has been argued that the issue of asylum seekers and refugees has emerged as an increasingly important aspect of social policy and debate in the past twenty years (Christie, 2003). It should be remembered that not all migrants are either asylum seekers or refugees, though they form a sizeable minority of migrant populations. Heated public and media debates have surrounded the policy decisions of international governments in relation to their management of asylum seekers and refugees. In Australia the arrangements put in place in 'holding centres' were the subject of national and international criticism, as were the arrangements in France, the UK, the Netherlands and Ireland among others.

Despite the debates, the trends of people seeking asylum from political, social or cultural persecution or indeed of economic migrants are obvious. These trends have at least forced questioning of traditional concepts of citizenship and social inclusion, exclusion, integration and cohesion. In an Irish context, the country has traditionally been characterised by a homogenous population and the trends have been more towards emigration than immigration.

Multiculturalism has been a relatively recent phenomenon that has brought social as well as health-promotion challenges. In Ireland it is estimated that immigration for the period April 2004–April 2005 was 70,000 (CSO, 2005). Of those, thirty-eight per cent were from the new EU states, with the majority from Poland and Lithuania. Twenty-seven per cent were Irish nationals returning. Twenty per cent were from the rest of the fifteen EU states, approximately three per cent from the US and thirteen per cent from the rest of the world. This trend has been consistent since at least 2000 (CSO, 2005). These figures suggest a pattern of economic migration as well as migration for other reasons.

However, economic migration suggests at least the possibility that those who migrate are coming from economic deprivation, suggesting some disadvantage at point of entry to the country in the first instance for some migrants. There is also strong evidence that migration is associated with a range of health-related difficulties, with differences evident between native populations and migrants in a variety of illness conditions including tuberculosis, HIV/AIDS and other sexually transmitted diseases, cardiovascular disorders, reproductive health, schizophrenia, depression, accidental injuries and psychosomatic illnesses (Carballo et al., 1998).

In addition to health inequalities, migration is also associated with a range of integration problems and issues of adjustment to new environments – at least in the first generation of migrants, where close family supports and a 'sense of community' has not been established (Wall and São José, 2004). This raises the issue of cultural identity, levels of separateness or integration and respect for difference. It also suggests a need to ensure that ethnic and cultural concerns are appropriately planned for and those plans implemented at policy and service levels. It has been argued that providing culturally competent and sensitive care can positively impact on health outcomes (Betchel *et al.*, 2000). Reinforcing this point, a study by Hjelm *et al.* (2005) pointed to quite divergent beliefs about what constituted 'health' between males from different ethnic backgrounds as well as what contributed to or influenced health.

HEALTH PROMOTION FOR ETHNIC AND CULTURAL HEALTH

Papandopoulos (1999) correctly argues that it is incorrect to make generalised assumptions about particular populations; however trends need to be heeded. At the heart of providing culturally appropriate care lies the requirement to understand and appreciate culture, which has been defined as:

> a patterned behavioural response that develops over time as a result of imprinting the mind through social and religious structures and intellectual and artistic manifestations. Culture is also the result of acquired mechanisms that may have innate influences but are primarily affected by internal and external environmental stimuli.
>
> (Newman Giger and Davidhizar, 2004:3)

As argued, the changing nature of the demographic profile in Ireland as well as Europe, which has been influenced by political, economic and social changes, is an important context in which to consider the role of health-promotion agents and approaches for planning and delivering culturally appropriate care. With both a common travel area across twenty-five European states and increasing inward migration from economically deprived or politically challenged countries outside the EU, the challenges to traditional service and policy norms become more pointed. In the context of migrant groups, Bhugra (2004) clearly points out the complexity of considering migration as a unitary concept.

Migration can clearly be forced or voluntary in nature and may occur among individuals or groups. While the process of migration is experienced in an unique manner, it impacts on individuals and communities differently (Bhugra, 2004). This clearly relates to the migrating population or individuals as well as the native populations. Moving into a new country and community has obvious challenges, but equally the difficulties associated with understanding and accepting differences by native populations as well as disruptions to the homogeneity or cohesiveness of local communities needs to be acknowledged. A clear concern relates to the level of integration with the host country or population or the level of distinctiveness. The central concern, therefore, is arriving at a balance between the protection and respect of cultural distinctiveness and ensuring the rights of particular populations while simultaneously supporting host communities.

In relation to ethnic groups, there is evidence that culture influences beliefs and behaviours related to health, although it would be wrong to assume that culture is the only factor that influences health behaviour (Papandopoulos, 1999). There is evidence that some lifestyle behaviours may be associated with ethnic difference (Rissel *et al.*, 2000). Making the healthier choice can be clearly associated with lifestyle opportunities for migrant populations. However, lifestyle choices should not be interpreted out of context.

Again, without making generalisations, many migrants are forced to leave their country of origin because of economic issues and are poor on arrival in their host country. Not alone will it be more difficult to make healthier choices when poor, but poverty can also make accessing health services for preventative and illness-management reasons difficult. Access to or use of appropriate health services for migrant populations or ethnic groups can be influenced by a range of issues. These might include experiences with official agencies prior to migration, language difficulties, lack of knowledge of the services available in the new country, lack of information or understanding of entitlements, cultural taboos or traditions and fear of authority or government agencies and services (Davidson *et al.*, 2004).

As argued earlier, health promotion involves the facilitation of individuals or groups in making healthier choices. Clearly, health-promotion agents can and should act at both individual and group levels to support ethnic groups in understanding the system in which they find themselves. At a very fundamental level, this will mean supporting them in understanding such issues as their entitlements and rights in order to make the healthier choices more easily.

Migrant populations and ethnic groups frequently seek out and live in existing discrete communities for support and cohesion. While the support available through these living arrangements is obvious and in many instances attractive, there is also a danger that segregation and ghettoisation may occur and lead to difficulties in their own right.

Developing economies such as the Irish economy need migrant labour for continued growth. Those in poorer countries need income and resources; those suffering from political or religious discrimination or persecution need asylum and refuge. These realities are now generally accepted. Therefore operating at a political and social level to understand and empower these groups is not just an option for health-promotion agents, but is an imperative. Acting as advocates for such groups is a necessary role that must be fulfilled to influence individual wellbeing as well as policy responses. Likewise mediating between host and migrant individuals and communities to foster understanding and acceptance of difference and similarities becomes a key issue in terms of implementing culturally sensitive and appropriate care as well as minimising and addressing health and social inequalities.

Promoting health and the Travelling community

Not all culturally distinct groups come from outside the country. This section will briefly consider the Travelling community in Ireland, which is recognised as a distinct minority group. Travellers are recognised as differing from the general population in terms of their culture, language, beliefs, values and lifestyle. The Equal Status Act (Government of Ireland, 2000:7) recognises their cultural distinctiveness in the following definition:

> Traveller community means the community of people who are commonly called travellers and who are identified (both by themselves and others) as people with a shared history, culture and traditions including, historically a nomadic way of life on the island of Ireland.

As a distinct cultural group they have been excluded and marginalised from the general population historically. According to the census of 2002 (CSO, 2004a) there were 24,000 Travellers nationally in 2002, the highest proportion of whom reside in the former Eastern Regional Health Authority area.

The Irish Traveller community also differs from general population in terms of health status. They have poorer health and shorter life expectancy. The shorter life expectancy is highlighted by the Central Statistics Office (CSO, 1998), who reported that only 1.5 per cent of Travellers are aged over sixty-five years. Life expectancy for male travellers is ten years less than their male counterparts in the general population. They have twice the risk of dying in any given year when compared with their counterparts in the settled community (Barry *et al.*, 1987). Traveller women also have shorter life expectancy, living on average twelve years less than other Irish women. (Barry *et al.*, 1987). This raises questions as to why this unique cultural group experiences such poor health status. A variety of factors potentially contributes to this health disadvantage of Travellers including social exclusion, racism, poverty, unemployment, educational disadvantage, accessibility and utilisation of services and health literacy.

Travellers have a higher than average birth rate. However, despite this, infant mortality and stillbirth rates are both more than double the national average (Barry *et al.*, 1987). In addition, sudden infant death syndrome (SIDS) was twelve times the national rate; with 8.8 deaths per 1,000 live births compared with 0.7 per 1,000 live births in settled communities (Irish Sudden Infant Death Association, 1999).

Half of the Traveller population is under fifteen years of age and seventy per cent is under twenty-five years of age (CSO, 1998). This suggests that Traveller youth could be a target group for health promotion. Travellers were identified as a key target group in the 1994 strategy *Shaping a Healthier Future* (DoHC, 1994:23) as one group where obvious health inequity needed to be addressed. It stipulated that:

> There is a particular obligation upon the health services to pay special attention to geographic areas or population groups (such as travellers) where the indicators of health status are below average.

A number of health-education and health-promotion programmes aimed at health gain for Travellers has been pursued in recent years. The success of those initiatives has been closely related to user involvement at all stages of the programme. Video and posters have been found to be the most effective media for conveying health messages to the Traveller population (DoHC, 2002). The cultural appropriateness of training materials and the importance of user involvement in the planning, delivery and evaluation of health-promotion interventions is an important consideration in promoting Traveller health.

However, as with other at-risk groups, while there is a strength in having focused health-promotion activity addressing the inequities and redressing imbalances in terms of opportunities, it is equally possible that focusing on high-risk groups can lead to victim blaming (Naidoo and Wills, 2000).

Travellers, as stated, have a high level of infant mortality. We could, for example, attribute this to poor utilisation of antenatal services, without exploring the factors that contribute to uptake of services and failing to consider the social and environmental determinants of health for Traveller babies. Likewise higher incidence of a range of health conditions could mistakenly be attributed in a very simplistic way to the nomadic ethos and living arrangements of the Travelling community. Failing to take account of lifestyle choices and traditions may result in settled communities 'forcing' their norms and values on such populations rather than designing and delivering services to take adequate account of difference. Attempts to force such groups to conform to the norms of dominant populations have been a feature of many cultures, but are inconsistent with the ethos and philosophy of health promotion. This highlights the importance of working with specific groups to identify their unique needs and delivering services in culturally appropriate ways.

Promoting the health of the mentally ill

The mentally ill, particularly those with serious and enduring mental illnesses, are identified as another marginalised group. We have already established that those with mental illness have poorer health than the general population. According to the UK Department of Health (2001) receiving a diagnosis of schizophrenia or bipolar disorder often results in a client's physical health being disregarded. Supporting this argument, in one of the more interesting comments in a recent Inspector of Mental Hospitals Report (DoHC, 2001c), the Inspector makes reference to the fact that psychiatric patients enjoy poorer health and have higher mortality than the general population, yet residents in mental health units have a poor level of physical health examination.

Equitable access to services was highlighted in Chapter 1 as a determinant of health. Persons with mental illness have a constitutional right to receive the same level of health care as the rest of the population. Indeed, Amnesty International (2003) called for the Irish government to acknowledge and respect the right of all people with mental illness in Ireland to the best available mental-health care.

Access to services, however, is but one of several factors that contribute to the health of the mentally ill. Research suggests that those with mental illness are more likely to engage in lifestyle behaviours that may further increase their risk of poor health (Davidson *et al.*, 2001a; Davidson *et al.*, 2001b; Brown *et al.*, 2000). As there is a paucity of Irish research in this area the studies discussed are international rather than national. Brown *et al.* (2000) prospectively surveyed the lifestyles of 140 people with schizophrenia with a group in the general population and found that their diet was unhealthy (higher in fat and lower in fibre than the reference population), they exercised less and had significantly higher levels of smoking than the reference population.

In the comparisons made, however, patients were not compared with individuals from similar social backgrounds, making it unclear to what extent poverty, housing and unemployment are causal factors rather than mental illness alone (Phelan, 2001). In an Australian study Davidson *et al.* (2001a) found that psychiatric outpatients (in a sample of 234) had a high prevalence of cardiovascular risk factors, (smoking, excess alcohol and salt intake, lack of exercise and obesity) which may account for the higher rate of cardiovascular mortality among those with mental illness. Studies of this nature highlight the need for promoting cardiovascular health in those with mental illness.

A higher prevalence of overweight and obesity among those with mental illness is reported in several studies (Bailey, 2002; Meyer, 2001; Wallace and Tennant, 1998; Beeber, 1988; Gopalaswamy and Morgan, 1985). Not eating a balanced diet, overeating, under-activity, lack of knowledge and weight gain as a side effect of psychotropic medication are suggested as causes of overweight and obesity in this group. As obesity increases the risk for lifestyle diseases, nutrition promotion is required in those with mental illness. In an Irish context there is increasing recognition that overweight and obesity is a serious health issue in some clients with mental illness. This awareness has led to the development of programmes such as Solutions for Wellness designed by a pharmaceutical company, which is currently available to mental-health service users. This programme, which has a nutrition component, was initially designed for clients who experienced weight gain on psychotropic medication and is now widely available to clients who wish to reduce weight.

Smoking is generally on the decline. However, a higher percentage of those with disorders such as schizophrenia smoke than the general population (Meadows *et al.*, 2001). High rates of smoking (forty-one per cent) are reported among individuals with any history of mental illness (Lasser *et al.*, 2000). Reported rates for those in institutional care are as high as seventy to seventy-four per cent (Meltzer *et al.*, 1996). Despite their high rates of smoking, those with serious mental-health problems do not seem to have been targeted for smoking-cessation interventions as strongly as other members of the community (Meadows *et al.*, 2001; SANE Australia, 2000). Indeed, despite the widely acclaimed success of the smoking ban in workplaces introduced nationally in 2004, mental-health units were excluded from this initiative. Nurses are generally regarded as having an important part to play in promoting smoking cessation; however, it appears that where there is a mental-health problem they may be less active in this role. In fact Cataldo (2001) suggests that mental-health nurses fail to consistently assess and treat tobacco use among service users.

A number of barriers to promoting smoking cessation in those with mental illness has been reported in the literature. Buchanan *et al.* (1994), for example, suggest that mental-health nurses might not view clients' smoking behaviour as a nursing issue. We would argue that such a perspective is contrary to the holistic view of clients that is central to health promotion. Others propose that nurses' own smoking status impacts on their view of whether patients should be encouraged to stop smoking or not (Dickens *et al.*, 2004; Clark *et al.*, 2004). The impact of nurses' smoking behaviour on their health-promotion role is discussed elsewhere in this book.

Perhaps mental-health nurses take cognisance of the positive aspects of smoking for those with mental illness reported in the literature. These include a calming effect, an amelioration of the positive symptoms of schizophrenia and a reduction in the side-effect profile of anti-psychotic medication (Spring *et al.*, 2003; Lawn *et al.*, 2002). Such a view fails to consider the negative impact of smoking on overall health. It has also been hypothesised that mental-health clinicians are reluctant to encourage smoking cessation because of the considerable stress and disability that clients are already experiencing because of their mental illness (Van Dongen and Fox, 1999). It has been argued that such rationalisation is ill-conceived and a subtle form of stigmatisation (Dalack and Glassman, 1992).

Promoting smoking cessation in those with mental illness may pose a challenge to health promoters. It is argued that those with specific disorders such as schizophrenia and depression associate greater advantages and reward value with cigarette smoking than do individuals without psychiatric disorders who smoke as heavily (Spring *et al.*, 2003). It is also argued that while this group is cognisant of the advantages and disadvantages of smoking, they consider that the advantages outweigh the drawbacks (Spring *et al.*, 2003). This is not to suggest that those with mental-health problems are not interested or motivated to give up smoking, rather it identifies a challenge that can be addressed by health promoters and smoking-cessation officers by tailoring interventions to individual needs rather that a one-size-fits-all approach to smoking cessation. It is our opinion that all those involved in caring for the mentally ill must collaboratively work towards promoting smoking cessation so that clients can make informed choices. The availability of supports such as nicotine replacement therapy to those in residential units and medical cardholders, plus the appointment of smoking cessation officers, are certainly steps in the right direction. The exemption of mental health units from the smoking ban is certainly contentious.

The empirical literature suggests that psychiatric diagnosis needs to be considered in assisting those with mental illness who want to quit smoking because of differences in perceptions and patterns of use (Lawn *et al.*, 2002). There have also been calls to modify cessation programmes to account for the cognitive, social and affective deficits of schizophrenia (Addington *et al.*, 1997). Evidence suggests that nursing interventions for smoking cessation are effective (Sarna, 1999; Wewers *et al.*, 1998). Mental-health professionals are in a unique position to promote smoking cessation in those with mental-health problems. Therefore it is important that mental-health nurses assess readiness to change, promote smoking cessation in those who wish to stop and educate others so that they are in an informed position to make change if desired.

Those with mental illness are identified in the literature as a high-risk group for HIV/AIDS and hepatitis. Davidson *et al.* (2001b), for example, investigated the risk factors for hepatitis and HIV among a group of 234 chronically mentally ill patients (seventy-nine per cent had a primary diagnosis of schizophrenia). They concluded that the prevalence of risk behaviour (unprotected sex, illicit drug use and needle sharing) among the study group indicated that people with chronic mental illness should be regarded as a high-risk group for HIV/AIDS and hepatitis C. In a review of the literature on HIV infection and schizophrenia, Gray *et al.* (2002) estimate that approximately two per cent (4000–5000) of people with schizophrenia in the UK are living with HIV/AIDS. Gray *et al.* (2002) conclude that HIV infection in those with schizophrenia is a serious but largely ignored part of the HIV epidemic and that those with schizophrenia should be considered an at-risk group who warrant special attention. While there are no figures to suggest that similar rates occur in Ireland and not wishing to stigmatise an already stigmatised group, a targeted health-promotion programme may help to save lives.

The literature suggests that sexuality is generally neglected in mental-health care (Earle, 2001; Park Dorsay and Forchuk, 1994). Historically, there was a tendency to desexualise those with mental illness or pathologise sexual expression (Cort *et al.*, 2001; Weinhardt *et al.*, 1997). UK research by Cort *et al.* (2001) which explored 122 community mental-health nurses' attitudes to and experience of sexuality-related issues in their work with people experiencing mental-health problems confirms sexuality as a relevant issue for community mental-health nurses. Cort *et al.* (2001) report an overwhelming affirmation by these mental-health nurses of people with mental-health problems as sexual beings. Yet a qualitative study of mental-health nurses conducted in one Irish county (Deasy, 2005) supports the view of Hyland *et al.* (2003) that the sexual health of those with mental illness continues to be ignored. Hyland *et al.* report that relatively few case managers inquired about the safe sexual practice of those with mental-health problems. Previously, Park Dorsay and Forchuk (1994) reported that nurses don't ask about sexual issues, are uncomfortable with the subject and do not consider the sexual domain in assessments. Patton *et al.* (1995) posit that many healthcare professionals feel uncomfortable in sexual-health education.

The Royal College of Nursing (RCN, 1996) underline that healthcare professionals do not provide adequate sexual health information and education to those with enduring mental illness. Lewis and Scott (1997) investigated the perceived sexual education needs of community-based clients with schizophrenia. They found that clients' description of their needs differed from the inferred needs of the investigators. This suggests the importance of needs assessment prior to planning intervention. It is also imperative that interventions are tailored to meet the needs and beliefs of those with mental illness. Likewise in Deasy's study (2005) Irish mental-health nurses reported a reluctance to normally enquire about the sexual health or practices of their clients or promote sexual health.

A number of barriers that inhibit health professionals from discussing sexual health have been identified in the literature. These include the belief that clients do not want to discuss sexual matters, that such a discussion may create distress, and a view that sexual concerns are of low priority (Cort *et al.* 2001 cites Cohen *et al.*, 1997; Risen, 1995; Kautz *et al.*, 1990). Educational deficit is also often cited as a constraint in relation to sexual-health promotion in nursing (Irwin, 1997). Research suggests that the sexual health education and training of practitioners is inadequate (Lewis and Bor, 1994; Mc Haffie, 1994). Sexual health is implicit in a holistic concept of health, therefore the sexual health of this group must be considered as an important part of their overall health.

Despite the benefits of exercise to physical and mental health, low levels of physical activity are reported internationally in clients with mental illness (Brown *et al.*, 2000; Davidson, 2001a). Additionally, Callaghan (2004:476) reports that exercise is seldom recognised in the care and treatment of mental-health problems and asserts 'exercise may be a neglected intervention in mental-health care'. In light of the benefits of exercise to health generally, mental-health professionals could play a key role in the integration of activity promotion into a holistic approach to health promotion with service users.

The research reviewed suggests that those with mental-health problems, particularly those with severe and enduring mental illness, may be engaging in lifestyle behaviours that contribute to their poor physical health status. This suggests a role for health promoters in promoting healthy lifestyles. However, it is important that health professionals do not engage in victim blaming by targeting the individual's behaviour without addressing the broader determinants of health. Therefore, health promotion with this population group must incorporate a holistic ontology.

Hyland *et al.* (2003) previously reported low self-esteem and lack of assertiveness as barriers to health promotion. The view that it is possible to promote health among all mental-health service users, regardless of diagnostic label (Deasy, 2005), concurs with the views of Maville and Huerta (2002:27) that 'everyone is capable of changing his behaviour'. While mental illness may pose a challenge to promoting health it is a challenge that can be overcome by tailoring interventions to meet the specific needs of those with mental illness.

Reducing the stigma associated with mental illness

Mental illness is one of the most stigmatised human conditions worldwide (Bloch and Singh, 1997). Stigma remains a huge problem for service users and is a barrier to accessing services (Tones and Green, 2004). Crehan (2001) cites research carried out in the former Western Health Board region of Ireland (Jones and Evans, 2001) which reported that the majority of people view mental health in a negative way and would only avail of mental-health services for extreme circumstances. Indeed the stigma often extends to those who work in the mental-health service and impacts on recruitment and retention (Wells *et al.*, 2000).

The Irish government in *Quality and Fairness* (DoHC 2001b) outlines the need to create greater public awareness and understanding of mental illness to reduce stigma. This reflects the importance of mental-health promotion. However, while planned and recommended by *Quality and Fairness* a specific strategy for mental health has not been published at time of writing. Given that the national strategy was published over five years ago, it is arguable that this reflects the low priority afforded to mental health from a public policy perspective. Service users have also called for the development of a national mental-health strategy (Mental Health Commission, 2004). We have argued elsewhere that while any strategy is welcome a single health strategy that places mental health at the core of health and wellbeing is essential.

Amnesty International (2003) calls for a public education and awareness campaign to counter the stigma of mental illness. More recently the Mental Health Commission (2004:113) report on stakeholder consultation on quality in mental-health services in Ireland highlights the challenge for the mental-health service in reducing the stigma associated with mental illness. The Mental Health Commission (2004) emphasises the need to educate the public 'not only about mental illness, but also about mental health'; a view also articulated by mental-health nurses (Deasy, 2005).

Section 2
Research and Health Promotion

7
Evidence-based Practice

Learning Outcomes:

On completion of this chapter the reader will be able to:

- understand the key aspects of evidence
- distinguish between evidence and the evidence-based movement
- discuss the contribution of the evidence-based movement to practice
- debate the value of ranking evidence in hierarchies.

INTRODUCTION AND CONTEXT

The term 'evidence-based practice' has gained increasing popularity in health-related care since it was first introduced in the latter part of the twentieth century. Such is its acceptance and currency in healthcare that it has been claimed to have 'evolved as the dominant theme of practice, policy, management and education within health services across the developed world' (Rycroft-Malone *et al.*, 2004:914). While such a claim may be somewhat arguable, there is little doubt that evidence-based practice and care are at least *one* of the dominant topics of discussion within healthcare nationally and internationally.

Evidence-based practice is generally understood to have had its genesis in the evidence-based medicine movement in the early 1980s (Bennett and Bennett, 2000). It has now been adopted and advocated by a wide range of other health-related professions, at least at official and policy levels. There is general consensus that decisions and interventions in healthcare should be based on sound evidence. Sackett *et al.* (1996) argue for evidence-based medicine as the 'conscientious, explicit and judicious use of current best evidence in making decisions about the care of individual patients'. This is also true for evidence-based practice in health promotion. However, a distinction needs to be drawn between the use of evidence in healthcare practice and the evidence-based movement. A brief examination of the definition of Sackett *et al.* (1996) implies moral, purposeful and judgment-based processes in the decision-making process and in itself there is little room for debate about the merits of adopting such a position. The evidence-based practice movement, however, evokes strong reactions from both those in favour of and those against its ethos and influence. Walker (2003) referred to *the movement* as being seduced by superlatives such as best practice, best evidence and best care (Walker, 2003). Indeed these terms are used interchangeably and are interrelated and an examination of the evolution of this movement will help explore the differences between the use of evidence and the evidence-based movement as a medium of change.

Cochrane (1979) argues that the economic agenda influenced the development of this movement. The basis of this position is that in situations of limited resources, choices in terms of expenditure must be made and therefore clear evidence of clinical effectiveness is vital to direct resources to areas where effectiveness can be proven. While there is a compelling economic and perhaps political argument as well as a certain logic in this position, there has been strong resistance among many healthcare professions to having their practice driven by resource agendas. Yet others embrace the concept as a political reality while more warmly espousing the concept as a worthy approach, driven by logic and the ideology of accountability within the context of best practice.

The language (or arguably rhetoric) of evidence-based practice has become an integral component of current professional debates within and between health professionals in the past two decades. The link with health economics remains evident in some of the more recent literature. In the context of nursing, for example, French argues that at least part of the attraction of evidence-based practice for administrators is 'its potential to rationalise costs in healthcare' (1999:72). Taylor, writing on behalf of the research committee of the British Dietetic Association, argues that 'a treatment must be as clinically effective as an alternative treatment of similar cost' (1998c:461). This reiterates the argument that existing and new investment in health services demands increasing justification.

Evidence-based practice is presented by its protagonists as an integrative concept based on the practitioner combining clinical judgment with the best evidence available at a point in time, combined with patient values and preference (Bennett and Bennett, 2000; Sackett *et al.*, 2000). However others consistently argue that evidence-based practice is a concept that is either unattainable or indeed unwelcome for practitioners and service users for a variety of reasons. Than *et al.* (2005:330), for example, argue that the term itself has become synonymous with 'systematic reviews and guidelines produced in "ivory towers" with questionable local applicability and relevance to the personal circumstances of many patients'. This type of damming indictment is not unusual in the professional literature and it raises the question of what is the perceived and real purpose or motivation in introducing evidence-based practice. Furthermore it raises the dilemma as to the type of evidence that constitutes the necessary evidence upon which to base professional judgments.

WHY EVIDENCE-BASED PRACTICE?

Evidence-based practice has become an apparently unstoppable force in health-service provision and an integral element of the philosophy and delivery of care of service organisations (Bury and Mead, 1998). The motivation seems to be driven by a number of factors and influences such as the growth of the consumer movement which has had a profound impact on medicine in particular and the health field more generally.

Healthcare professions such as medicine have traditionally dominated health-service provision and the high status afforded them places them in a position to lead service policy and provision. This expert-led dominance remained generally unchallenged until the evolution of the consumer movement. The vastly increased availability of and accessibility to information has meant that a considerably greater demand for accountability has been placed on health-service providers, with assumptions of expertise being less likely to be accepted unquestioningly by informed consumers. This consumer-based approach is of course embedded in the Universal Declaration of Human Rights (United Nations, 1948), which identifies health as one of our fundamental human rights as opposed to a privilege. Thus the widespread acceptance of evidence-based practice is arguably no more than an alternative means of assuring quality care through research-based practice.

Evidenced-based practice is possibly the most important force committed to reshaping both thinking and practice in biomedicine (Mykhalovskiy and Weir, 2004). Internationally and nationally, evidence-based practice is increasingly underpinning health strategies and policies (McKenna *et al.*, 2002; DoHC, 2001b).

Accountability is one of the cornerstones upon which evidence-based practice is built. In many ways, within healthcare professions accountability was traditionally understood to be associated with outcomes, but was not particularly concerned with cost and resources. In other words, accountability tended to be interpreted in terms of the patient's getting well, with less emphasis being placed on comparative approaches or indeed on cost. During the 1980s and 1990s when evidence-based practice was evolving as the new paradigm for practice in medicine and related professions, the international (at least in the Western world) economic and political climates were conducive to greater economic and public accountability in service provision.

Legal accountability is another factor in the development of this movement. Increased levels of litigation have forced practitioners to be more conscious of current trends and best practice. The association between legal accountability and evidence-based practice has contributed in some measure to opposition towards the evidence-based movement.

WHAT CONSTITUTES EVIDENCE?

Evidence within medicine has traditionally been drawn from a biomedical scientific positivist tradition. Evidence, within this understanding, would essentially constitute research evidence drawn from research activity from positivist scientific traditions. The types of research most valued in positivist traditions tend to be those characterised by objectivity such as experiments and randomised control trials. One of the most contentious debates associated with the evidence-based practice movement is that *evidence* and *research* have tended to be used synonymously.

Evidence has a number of possible meanings, depending on context and use. For example, in the presentation of a model of evidence in healthcare, Upshur draws on a number of sources to argue that 'evidence is an observation, fact or organised body of information, offered to support or justify inferences or beliefs in the demonstration of some proposition or matter at issue' (2000:93). What is notable here is that this definition does not propose a hierarchical ordering of levels of evidence. However, in practice certain forms of evidence are prioritised over others. The hierarchies of evidence that are presented as being most valid tend to favour research-based evidence with a rank order normally favouring systematic reviews, randomised controlled trials and experiments over qualitative findings.

The traditions of medicine are deeply rooted in empiricism and as a consequence its research evidence is generally presented by its proponents and understood by others to be more generalisable and 'sound' than other research traditions. However, Upshur points out that medical evidence rarely achieves levels of absolute certainty, but rather is 'provisional, defeasible, emergent, incomplete, constrained, collective and asymmetric' (2000:93). It is in that context that evidence needs to be considered, evaluated and used.

Consistent theorists in fields such as nursing have challenged the supremacy of knowledge drawn from positivist traditions. Carper (1978) argues that diverse 'ways of knowing' exist, suggesting a variety of forms of evidence that can contribute to our knowledge base and on which we can base our actions. She argues that, in addition to empirical ways of knowing (which have traditionally been highly valued), we also draw on ethical or moral ways of knowing, aesthetics and personal experience among others. Research that incorporates the multiple ways of knowing that practitioners employ every day must also be understood to constitute valid and legitimate evidence.

INCORPORATING EVIDENCE INTO PRACTICE

There is little doubt that the evidence-based practice movement is central to health-service agendas internationally. There is evidence of some polarisation between two opposing groups. One group supports the value of this movement and articulates the benefits for the public or any of the healthcare professions of evidence-based practice, and the other group views the movement as one that is attempting to colonise healthcare services and vehemently opposes the evidence-based practice movement, though not necessarily the use of evidence.

One of the principal and most consistent themes among those who oppose evidence-based practice as a movement is the perception that autonomous practice and reliance on clinical judgment is undervalued. Perhaps more explicitly, some practitioners fear the imposition of an ideology of practice grounded in the positivist tradition and which originated in epidemiology, which is perceived to draw on the reductionist ethos and traditions of biological medicine. This could be interpreted as reinforcing the dominance of a principally reductionist approach in healthcare that fails to give due regard to the values, traditions and contributions of alternative and arguably more holistic and socially inclusive perspectives on health.

Within that context there are a number of immediate factors that need to be considered with regard to evidence-based practice, including the following:

The nature and quality of the evidence

It is not only the sources of evidence that need to be considered; the quality of the evidence available is also important. Likewise, evidence should not be interpreted solely as research evidence, although clearly research evidence is one extremely important type of evidence.

The skills of the healthcare personnel in generating, interpreting, applying and evaluating evidence

Resistance to evidence-based practice has been influenced by the perception that professional judgments made by practitioners are of less value than 'imposed' models of evidence. However, clinical judgment is a vital element of evidence-based practice. Therefore, healthcare personnel must have the training, skill and ongoing opportunity to contribute to the generation of knowledge. Traditionally not all healthcare practitioners were involved in primary research or evidence generation. However, it is also arguable that they are best positioned to be the generators of the evidence needed to inform practice. Therefore a reconceptualisation of the part that research plays within the role of the health professional is necessary. All healthcare practitioners need adequate skills to generate, interpret and apply evidence in practice and must also have the ability to evaluate its effectiveness.

The accessibility of findings

One of the consistent reasons provided by healthcare practitioners for the under-utilisation of evidence in practice relates to the accessibility of current research. The problem lies more in the lack of the technical language, skills and/or motivation to comprehend findings rather than the unavailability of literature, databases and library resources. Healthcare staff are more likely to rely on protocols and guidelines than primary research sources (Gerrish and Clayton, 2004).

Professional development in supporting healthcare practitioners in becoming confident in the reading and integration of research into their practice is necessary.

Organisational support and culture

One of the key factors in incorporating an ethos of evidence-based practice is the organisational commitment to basing practice on evidence and the existence of a culture of excellence. Practical and moral support within organisations is important for the integration of evidence-based practice. Management understanding of the time needed to source, understand, review and implement evidence is imperative.

Cobban (2004) points out that there are a number of assumptions on which evidence-based practice is predicated that are attractive to key stakeholders in healthcare. These include the assumptions that evidence-based practice is efficient, current, based on sound evidence and that it may narrow the 'theory–practice gap'. While evidence-based practice may impact on effectiveness of interventions and health and social outcomes, effectiveness frequently comes with a 'cost'. The 'cost' might include investment in the provision of appropriate training, support and time. It cannot be automatically assumed that healthcare staff have the skills or expertise to access, comprehend or use the evidence available, so training becomes an important issue. The complexity of individual, operational, organisational and professional relationships impacts on the introduction or application of evidence-based practice within the workplace. So while there may well be individual willingness or resistance to commit to evidence-based practice, a myriad of factors must be managed within organisations for the approach to be effective (Rycroft-Malone *et al.*, 2004).

One of the more pragmatic barriers that is frequently cited is 'time' (Gerrish and Clayton, 2004). Thus time is clearly a factor for consideration within organisations that claim to value evidence and support evidence-based practice. All concerned must be reassured that evidence-based practice is being engaged in as a means to enhance the process, experience and outcomes of care, rather than a form of overt or covert control. This is also an issue that emerges in the literature as a concern among those who question the evidence-based practice movement – though not necessarily the use of evidence itself (Winch *et al.*, 2002; Clarke, 1999).

8
Research Paradigms

Learning Outcomes:

On completion of this chapter the reader will be able to:
* understand the differing paradigms within health research
* critically debate differences between key paradigms such as those between positivist and naturalistic paradigms
* discuss the key research characteristics associated with differing paradigms.

INTRODUCTION

In Chapter 7 the issue of the nature of knowledge and different ways of knowing and their relative importance and applicability is explored. Indeed that chapter also argues that in health-related areas of practice, scientific knowledge drawn almost exclusively from a positivist tradition has traditionally been more highly regarded and firmly established as being more credible than other forms of knowledge. This implies that there are different traditions associated with knowledge generation and testing. If we assume that research is primarily concerned with the generation and testing of knowledge, then understanding the various research paradigms becomes an integral element of successful research. If research is to adequately generate and address topics or questions in a credible manner, there must be an obvious, consistent and coherent methodological approach. This chapter will explore the different research paradigms and their relationships with health promotion.

Research design is frequently described in a dichotomous manner with a distinction drawn between quantitative and qualitative methods. However, when such descriptions are used, it is arguable that they refer to the type of data collected, rather than provide an explanation of the research approach and the philosophical assumptions underpinning the choice.

The notion of 'paradigm' can be described as the ways in which scientific communities agree on their understanding of reality and the means by which reality might be understood through research (Clark, 1998). Another way of describing 'paradigm' may be as a scientific worldview or philosophy. The term 'research approach' refers to the type of research orientation associated with a particular paradigm and 'methods' refers to the types of techniques or means by which the research is undertaken (Haase and Taylor Myers, 1998).

Research is designed and undertaken within particular contexts and with differing driving forces or influences. For example the evidence-based practice movement has been a key driving force for the promotion of research in the healthcare field. Research activity (including design and scope) is also influenced by the types of funding available, the source of funding, and by professional hierarchies and agendas with regard to what actually constitutes legitimate research.

However, we would argue that at a more fundamental level it is more important that research is driven by coherent philosophical perspectives. Researchers should make their research decisions based on clear ontological assumptions (how we understand reality) and epistemological assumptions (how we understand the nature of knowledge). The key requirement of 'good research' is that there is a consistency between the choice of paradigms and the area of research. In other words, there must be clear evidence of a link between the research topic, the philosophical assumptions underpinning the paradigm and the methods chosen.

Traditionally healthcare practice and professional development have been based on the premise that positivistic scientific knowledge is superior to practice knowledge. This form of knowledge has been perceived as synonymous with, and based on, traditions, rituals and/or instinct and thus less legitimate. Scientific knowledge has been assumed to be value-free, generalisable, universal and objective. Such scientific knowledge has been the cornerstone of the development and pre-eminence of medicine within the healthcare field. The perspective of scientific knowledge and more specifically, the medical model, is highly respected and well established and has enjoyed a long-standing dominance in health discourse. However, other perspectives have challenged that dominance, particularly throughout the middle to latter half of the twentieth century. There have been growing challenges to the perceived objectivity and universality of scientific knowledge (at least from positivist traditions). It has been argued that positivistic scientific knowledge is potentially contextual, political, provisional and bound within temporal considerations. It is also limited by and through the use of language, particularly as language is constantly changing and is socially constructed (Bjornsdottir, 2001).

There is now little disagreement that much 'health' related activity, including health promotion, falls into a category of 'social science' as opposed to 'natural science'. Medicine in particular draws significant portions of its knowledge base from the natural sciences. The natural sciences, perhaps led by physics, have been dominated by the traditions of positivism. Social sciences are most associated with fields such as psychology, sociology, nursing, midwifery and education. Ironically, social scientists tended to follow and accept some of the main arguments about positivist-based knowledge. This might be partly explained by a desire to emulate the achievements, success, respect and acceptance of the natural sciences (Hughes and Sharrock, 1997).

Philosophers such as Kuhn have furthered the debate regarding the presumed dominant authority of positivist-based scientific knowledge. Kuhn (1970) argued that scientists developed plausible explanations of the world and relationships because they presented coherent arguments and that the means by which they arrived at their conclusions were structured and transparent. However, he argued that such arguments were transient in many instances and only accepted until challenged and/or new 'truths' emerged.

The latter half of the twentieth century saw the emergence of two other key research paradigms (naturalism and critical theory) that challenged the dominance of positivism in health and social sciences. The following sections will consider the key features of these three paradigms. The order in which they are presented should not be taken as a hierarchical ordering, but as positivist research paradigms have been in existence for the longest period, we believe that this is the most logical point of departure for any discussion of research paradigms.

POSITIVIST RESEARCH

The positivist research tradition is one that is deeply rooted in principles of observation, objectivity, detachment, control and certainty. Positivism has its origins in the natural sciences and places a high value on both logic and sensory experience. In addition to the natural sciences it has been the dominant paradigm within the social sciences (Guba, 1990), at least until fairly recent times. The key ontological assumptions of the positivist tradition are that reality is 'external' to the individual researcher. It presumes that the world or phenomena operate according to natural laws and that the principal function of research is to predict and control natural phenomena.

From an epistemological perspective, positivism assumes that the key function of research is to study phenomena as they exist, in an objective manner and without attempting to influence how things are within the world. This implies objectivity and adopting a neutral stance as an observer. It also means that researchers from a positivist tradition do not allow personal beliefs, biases or values to interfere with the objective nature of research.

Methodologically, research in the positivist tradition will normally be driven or guided either by an *a priori* theoretical position or by a particular hypothesis. Once the theory or hypothesis is formulated and made explicit, then it may be tested. This perspective forms the basis of the research approach within this tradition. Within this approach, it is then assumed that anything that might possibly interfere with the objective nature of the research can and should be controlled for. Both the establishment of the investigation and the conduct of the research should be characterised by a rigorous approach and based on these conditions. It is normally assumed that the aim of engaging in such research is that findings should be generalisable to wider populations.

Some of the key aims of positivist research are to discover *how* and *why* the world and phenomena within the world are the way they are. In that sense, research in this tradition allows researchers to describe, explain and/or predict phenomena. Therefore, experimentation is central to positivist research and is most associated with *experimental* or *quasi-experimental* designs.

Positivist paradigms and experimental research are mostly associated with laboratory settings, where the conditions and settings can be controlled. However, researchers in the social sciences normally study human beings in social situations rather than laboratory settings. As such they cannot completely control for all factors in individuals' environments that may influence the research process or outcomes. Where the researcher is the observer of social phenomena, positivism requires the researcher to effectively 'look in' on the social arrangements, relationships or phenomena under investigation as an independent and objective observer. Adopting such a stance is referred to as adopting an 'etic' (independent and objective) position and is one of the key facets of positivist research in the social sciences.

It should also be remembered that positivist research requires a logical, questioning and systematic approach. Research undertaken within this paradigm is founded on curiosity and the approach will be characterised by its attention to detail and its level of organisation and objectivity. Positivist research prides itself in its level of dispassionate critique, lack of bias and its rigour. These are effectively the traits that will characterise the positivist researcher. These characteristics imply a level of detachment that is also a hallmark of a classic positivist approach. This requires researchers to be neutral observers and recorders, who report findings that are free from any cultural, social, or experiential bias (Phillips, 1990). This approach, which can be described as 'empirical', is based on the belief that knowledge is developed or exposed through the use of systematic approaches, carefully observing and cataloguing phenomena, which in turn contributes to the discovery of infallible and universal laws (Clark, 1998).

The presumption of infallibility and universality of knowledge has long been disputed, other than in very particular and limited cases (for example, it is generally agreed that once an individual is born, death is inevitable). The limitations to the infallibility and the universal nature of positivist-based scientific 'truth' have been acknowledged by those who subscribe to the empirical research principles in more recent times. However the principles of objectivity, detachment, attention to detail and structure, rigour and logic are still considered important. In that sense, many researchers who subscribe to these principles and standards could be said to be influenced by the 'postpositivist' movement, which acknowledges the presence and indeed appropriateness of the measurement of unobservable phenomena, at least in their capacity to explain the functioning of observable phenomena. Likewise, researchers who subscribe to a postpositivist perspective acknowledge the conditionality and contingent nature of data, rather than the earlier emphasis on absolute certainty, or the universal application of laws and infallibility.

Indeed in the mid-1970s, both the relevance and dominance of one of the core tenets of positivist research – hypothesis testing – was called into question. It was argued that 'the time has come to exorcise the null hypothesis', (Cronbach, 1975:124). This was argued on the basis that primary concentration on affirming or refuting the null hypothesis, while important in itself, could miss factors that were not statistically significant.

NATURALISTIC RESEARCH

At the beginning of this chapter we argued that health-related research has been strongly influenced by the traditions of positivism in its broadest sense. However, since at least the middle of the twentieth century this dominance has been challenged. This has occurred for a variety of reasons, particularly the evolution of a variety of professions as distinct academic disciplines. Many of these new academic disciplines, principally in the social sciences such as nursing, midwifery and occupational therapy, recognise the value of positivism, but have also embraced naturalistic or critical-theoretic research methodologies. Indeed some of these disciplines actively promote these approaches as ones that are more appropriate to the illumination of practice-based knowledge.

Research methods within naturalistic paradigms are frequently described as qualitative methods, but we suggest that this categorisation is somewhat misleading as the term 'qualitative' more accurately refers to the data and collection processes rather than the approach itself. It is more appropriate to consider the overall approach as 'naturalistic' although it is acknowledged that the terms are frequently used interchangeably.

Naturalistic approaches are driven by a belief that people cannot be considered outside the context of their own worlds and therefore their experiences cannot be understood in total objectivity. This means that there are multiple interpretations of reality and the notion of one universal truth or absolute certainty is an anathema to this understanding of reality. Therefore, epistemologically, naturalistic studies differ from positivist ones in that they generally attempt to describe and explain the world from the perspective of the individual rather than from the sole perspective of the researcher, and they do not attempt to control or manipulate variables. The research process is effectively inductive and the researcher is understood to be someone who enters the world of the participants and maps that world. Within the mapping process, the researcher is seen as operating from one of two broad perspectives, namely the interpretivist and the constructivist perspectives.

These two perspectives reflect the divergent positions taken by two of the key theorists who have been hugely influential in naturalistic research, namely Edmund Husserl and Martin Heidegger. Somewhat similarly to those from positivist traditions, interpretivists claim that their findings can be judged with a level of objectivity because they engage in a process referred to as 'bracketing'. They assume that while they enter the social world of others, which in itself is unique, that reality is open to representation and interpretation. Bracketing is a process whereby interpretivist researchers try to put to one side past experiences, personal assumptions, beliefs and values. In practice, within some research methods this would mean, for example, not making reference to literature around a topic area prior to data collection so that judgments or descriptions are not unduly influenced.

In contrast, constructivists adopt what is referred to as an 'emic' position in research. They do not see themselves as being detached from the research process or the world of the participants. Instead they engage with them as partners in the construction of an account of phenomena. Constructivist researchers assume that it is impossible to completely bracket out experiences, values or beliefs, and that their key function is to construct accounts of reality in partnership with their research participants.

Naturalistic approaches are most associated with grounded theory, Husserlian and Hermeneutic phenomenology, ethnography and case studies. Issues associated with specific approaches will be addressed separately in their relevant sections.

9
Critical Theory

Learning Outcomes:

On completion of this chapter the reader will be able to:

* understand the principles of critical theory
* debate the contribution of critical theory to health-promotion research activity.

INTRODUCTION

The term critical theory emerged from the Frankfurt School (a research institute for social research in Frankfurt, Germany) in the 1930s. Horkheimer was the first to define critical theory as a form of theory generation that is concerned with the improvement of society by focusing on critique of current social formations and the construction of society. The key distinction of this approach is that it is essentially political in that it is seen as a stimulus for action and change.

Members of the Frankfurt School argued that there were significant limitations inherent in existing research approaches and argued that the focus of research should be practical, based on critique, and that prioritisation of the need for change should be implicit within the research. A central tenet of critical theory is 'emancipation'. Horkheimer (1982:244) argues that the purpose of critical theory is to promote the emancipation of people and to 'liberate human beings from all the circumstances that enslave them'. This concept of enslavement is clearly related to power relationships and how these are constituted within society.

Critical theorists would argue that power is actively constituted in the relationships that people engage in on a daily basis. Hierarchical power relationships have become synonymous with organisations and systems, such as education, health, economics and politics, within many, if not all societies. Such hierarchical systems can lead to a sense of disenfranchisement for many within society. Critical theorists argue that those who hold power to make political and economic decisions within society constitute a social 'elite' and the decisions they make reinforce dominant social formations of inequality for the benefit of these same elites. A critical theoretic approach focuses specifically on elites, an exploration of how power is negatively used for the benefit of social elitism and the cost of these social constructs to those who are less powerful or marginalised within society. Key questions might relate to how our health system is structured and how it may contribute to or reinforce social inequality rather than actively seeking to redress it.

Critical theory represents a broad school of thought that involves uncovering the nature of power relationships within a given society, and that also seeks through its inquiries to help emancipate members of the culture from the many forms of oppressions that operate within it (Gall, Borg and Gall 1999:361).

Thus research which holds at its core the values of emancipation, empowerment and critical engagement while seeking to address oppression in its many forms may be considered to rest within the umbrella of critical theory. According to Horkheimer (1982) the criteria for critical theory are three-fold. It must be explanatory, practical and normative. In other words it must explain what is wrong with current society, identify the factors needed to change it and provide norms for criticism and achievable practical goals for social transformation (Bohman, 2005). In its broadest sense the work of Michel Foucault and Pierre Bourdieu as well as feminism, critical race theory, post-colonial critique, queer theory can also be termed critical theory. Thus it can be argued that the intent of critical theoretic research is in essence political in that it seeks a more democratic and egalitarian society.

CRITICAL THEORY AND HEALTH-PROMOTION RESEARCH

In considering the relevance of critical theory for health-promotion research, it might be useful to consider the concepts of emancipation and empowerment. Emancipation is central to the Frankfurt School's thinking. Conceptually this is not at significant variance from the notion of empowerment, which in itself is outlined in the Ottawa Charter (WHO, 1986) as a core principle of health-promotion practice. In order to support health-promotion practitioners in empowering clients and communities, research which places priority on the critique of dominant ideologies and their impact on individual client and population health is necessary.

Ideology can be understood as 'the values and practices emanating from particular dominant groups [and] is the means by which powerful groups promote and legitimate their particular sectoral interests at the expense of disempowered groups' (Cohen, Manion and Morrison, 2000:30). Critique of ideologies that permeate both the health services and professions is necessary to identify the causes of health inequalities. However, the critique must go further than identification in that it must also lead to the creation of alternative ideologies of health practice that are grounded in democracy. In other words, in the context of health services, the research endeavour seeks to redress both the cause and practice of health inequality. Thus a critical theoretic approach to health-promotion research would foster a process of ideology critique that is practical and motivated towards social change.

Habermas (1972) advocates a critical theoretic approach to ideology critique in order to identify the vested interests at work that maintain a system of disempowerment. He states that this ideological critique can be carried out in four stages. The first stage requires an assessment of the current situation. The second stage looks to the causes behind what is happening including analysis of the power and legitimacy of the current situation. Stage three includes engaging in action in order to move towards more democratic principles, and finally stage four requires reflection and evaluation of the new situation created as a result of the action.

For example, health-promotion research in the area of health inequalities within a critical theoretic research approach would require an in-depth look at current inequalities, analysis of the ideologies that underpin the reproduction of social inequalities, engagement in planning and implementation of action to address these inequalities and finally evaluation of the process. One can see the philosophical similarities to the principles of action research in the focus on critical analysis and improvement towards a better social order. Thus in a critical theoretic approach research is not simply an objective observation of reality but is motivated by a specific agenda of critical analysis and social change.

Questions at the core of a critical theoretic approach are of the kind, 'research in whose interests' (Usher, 1996). Thus the research agenda within critical theory is emancipatory but equally the process must be empowering of research participants. Thus the goal and the process are motivated by the same agenda – emancipation. In the area of health research from a critical perspective the focus is also placed on the politics of how power and wealth are unequally distributed within society and the impact this has on population health. Given that advocacy, capacity building and equity are key principles in the promotion of health as outlined by the World Health Organization (WHO, 1986). Critical theory clearly has its place in health-promotion research. To date it is an approach not widely used within this field, but the increasing national awareness of health inequalities as heavily influenced by geographical location and socioeconomic background in Ireland are pointing to the need for critical analysis of the legitimacy of policy development and national strategic planning. A critical theoretic approach could provide an excellent framework within which to formulate such critique in order to employ research as an effective strategy for change.

10
Phenomenology

Learning Outcomes:

On completion of this chapter the reader will be able to:

- understand the principles of phenomenology
- distinguish between phenomenology as a philosophy and as a research approach
- discuss the differing traditions within phenomenology
- debate the use of phenomenology in health-promotion research activity.

INTRODUCTION

Phenomenological research has its origins in the work of mainland European philosophers, especially those from Germany, France, Holland and Belgium. However, phenomenology as a research approach remained relatively unknown in English-speaking countries for a considerable period (Thomas, 2005). Edmund Husserl (1859–1938) is generally credited as the founder of phenomenology. Ironically, Husserl, who was a mathematician, is considered as the founder of an approach which is seen as being the antithesis of empirical approaches to understanding, in which the laws of mathematical science are central.

PHENOMENOLOGY AS A PHILOSOPHY

Phenomenology, as Husserl saw it, was concerned with understanding the meaning of events or phenomena as well as the essence of phenomena. Husserl argued that in order to understand essential meaning, individuals had to put aside their usual means of understanding. He argued that because many phenomena exist in our world with us, we may take them for granted. In order that we could understand the essence of their meaning, Husserl argued that we must put aside this 'taken for granted' understanding and adopt a particular attitude, which can be referred to as a 'phenomenological attitude'. When such an approach is adopted, then we can seek out the essential traits and characteristics of the phenomenon and arrive at a deep understanding of its true meaning.

This notion of meaning is central to all forms of phenomenological endeavour and is a prominent feature of all traditions within the phenomenological 'family'. This concept of phenomenology as a 'family' or a movement as originally described by Spielberg (1960) is also an important issue in understanding and describing phenomenology. For example, Cohen (1987) identifies three particular phases in the evolution of phenomenology, namely the preparatory phase, the German phase and the French phase. While the geographic division is a useful description, it is perhaps more interesting that phenomenology can be understood as an evolving and dynamic movement. While Edmund Husserl, as argued, is generally understood to be the founder of phenomenology, Cohen argues that Husserl's work further developed the work of Franz Brentano (1838–1917) and Carl Stumpf (1848–1936). Stumpf was a student of Brentano and is generally credited with demonstrating that phenomenological approaches adhere to the principles of scientific rigour.

While Husserl built on the earlier work of those with whom he studied – Brentano and Stumpf (Cohen,1987) – and has remained a dominant figure in the field of phenomenology, it is also interesting that one of his students, Martin Heidegger (1889–1976) subsequently emerged as a central figure in phenomenology. The third 'phase' as described by Cohen (1987) refers to the influence of French philosophers such as Gabriel Marcel (1889–1973), Jean Paul Sartre (1905–80) and Maurice Merleau-Ponty (1908–60). Perhaps the most important issue to understand is that phenomenology is a dynamic and evolving philosophy.

PHENOMENOLOGY AS A SCIENTIFIC METHOD

Phenomenology is both a philosophical understanding and a research approach. From a research perspective, it is an approach that attempts to understand phenomena, or the appearance of things, in which phenomenological 'intuiting' is understood as being the yardstick against which knowledge is gauged. Intuiting, in a phenomenological sense, involves the use of logic to arrive at an insight of phenomena. Likewise conclusions or findings in phenomenological research are not based on first impressions, but on careful analysis of reports of phenomena.

It can be argued that intuiting is the cornerstone of phenomenological approaches to research. However, two of the key figures within the phenomenological movement, namely Husserl and Heidegger, differ in their interpretation of this and related concepts. This has led to the evolution of two distinct and ironically dichotomous traditions within phenomenological research, referred to as interpretivism and constructivism.

We would argue that these traditions have influenced research practices that have drawn on the philosophical understandings of phenomenology and that there are core concepts that run through the different traditions. One of the shortcomings of phenomenological researchers is that they have failed to clearly describe or define phenomenological research methods *per se*, but rather their descriptions are more concerned with the philosophy (Sadala and de Camargo Ferreira Adorno, 2002). In that sense, methods of undertaking phenomenological research are to be found implicitly rather than explicitly throughout the work of the central figures in phenomenology. Indeed, Johnson (2000) argues that while key figures such as Heidegger never intended the development of a research method as such in their work, methodological approaches can be inferred through their work.

CORE CONCEPTS OF PHENOMENOLOGY AS RELATED TO PHENOMENOLOGICAL RESEARCH

Intentionality of consciousness

Intentionality is generally seen as being at the core of phenomenology and phenomenological research. In somewhat simplistic terms it may be described as the manner in which the consciousness is directed towards an object (Cohen, 1987), or perhaps more precisely as the 'direction of consciousness towards understanding the world' (Sadala and de Camargo Ferreira Adorno, 2002). The implication from this understanding is that phenomenology understands existence as being integrated and holistic in that intentionality of consciousness must be directed towards something within the world and as such, consciousness and the world are interdependent for meaning to be possible.

Therefore, the notion of intentionality of consciousness is a clear distinguishing characteristic between phenomenological research and positivism. Positivism, with its roots in Cartesian dualism, believes in the separation, or at least separate existence, of mind and body. Phenomenological traditions argue that this is not possible. Indeed Heidegger argued that humans could not be seen as 'subjects' in a reductionist way, but rather described people as 'being-in-the-world'. This notion of integration between consciousness, intentionality and 'the world' which includes both concrete and abstract world experiences is central to the function or role of researchers operating within a phenomenological tradition. This has been aptly described by Sadala and de Camargo Ferreira Adorno (2002:283) who argue that the role of the phenomenological researcher 'is to analyse the intentional experiences of consciousness in order to perceive how a phenomenon is given meaning and to arrive at its essence'.

Phenomenological intuiting

Phenomenological intuiting should not be confused with the concept of intuition. Intuition can be seen as having both a 'lay' and a 'professional' meaning. In its everyday sense, operating on intuition can be understood as acting or frequently reacting to situations in ways that are characterised by insights or actions that are at very least difficult to explain and not necessarily based on known evidence. In some professional writings, intuition is explained in terms of dissonance or subconscious associations between experience and cognition. In the context of nursing, Benner and Tanner (1987:23) describe intuition as involving an 'understanding without rationale' and they associate this concept with expertise in professional practice. They suggest that intuition is virtually an innate quality of the practitioner who has developed to the level of 'expert' practice and is based mainly on the fact that such practitioners are 'operating from a deep understanding of the total situation' (Benner, 1984:32). While this clearly suggests an integration of cognitive processes through experience and therefore 'drawing' on experience from life, it could also be interpreted as being an inherent quality rather than a conscious process. This should not be confused with phenomenological intuiting.

Cohen (1987) described phenomenological intuiting as both the 'test of all knowledge' and an activity that 'involves logical insight based on careful consideration of representative examples' (Cohen, 1987:31). This suggests that phenomenological intuiting is a process aimed at arriving at knowledge by adopting a detailed and structured approach. This assertion suggests that it is possible to transform or transpose the principles of phenomenology from a philosophical perspective to a research approach, despite the arguments that this may never have been the direct intention of some of the founding fathers of phenomenology.

Phenomenological reduction

In the same way that terms such as intentionality of consciousness have specific meaning in phenomenology, reduction in the phenomenological sense should not be mistaken for reductionism. Husserl originally introduced this term and drew on the Greek word 'epoche' to describe his intent. He argued that when arriving at an essence of meaning, it was vital to remove any assumptions about the phenomenon under consideration through a process of retrogression.

Reduction, from a Husserlian perspective, means that no position is taken in relation to an experience. In such circumstances, it is assumed that prejudices or preconceptions cannot interfere with reality. Merleau-Ponty (1962) described this as a phenomenological device that allows for discovery of the 'life-world'. It is assumed that the effect of this device is that the reduction results in the individual assuming the position of a 'disinterested observer'. While this is a useful description, the idea of being a disinterested observer could also be misinterpreted. Disinterested observation must be understood within the overall purpose of reduction. The aim of the reduction is to achieve either a pre-reflexive state or a level of primitive contact with the world as we actually experience it without the added complexity of reflection and conceptualisation of the world. The core aim of the reduction is to focus on the essence of meaning of the experience and the uniqueness of that experience.

While we have used the terms 'technique', 'stance' and 'device' to describe reduction, it is perhaps more accurate to describe it as a level of attentiveness. It does not describe a prescribed procedure, but it can be achieved through particular routes. Language is seen as the principal medium through which meaning may be accessed and ultimately made intelligible; both the spoken word and writing are important to phenomenological inquiry. Reduction requires reflective attentiveness as a virtual attribute as opposed to a method if meaning is to be achieved.

Husserlian phenomenology introduced the concept of 'bracketing' to reflect the state of 'epoche', which was seen as a requirement for phenomenological inquiry. Jasper, (1994:311) described this process as the 'deliberate examination by researchers of their own beliefs about a phenomenon and the temporary suspension of these'.

Bracketing emerged as one of the central distinctions between Husserlian and Heideggerian phenomenology, with Heidegger (1962) refuting the contention that it is possible to 'bracket' previous experiences, beliefs or preconceptions. He argued that this was inconsistent with the understanding of individuals 'being-in-the-world'. In such an integrated state, it was believed by Heidegger and his followers that it is impossible to achieve a state of separation between the individual and the world. Therefore assumptions, beliefs, and values could not be left aside. This in turn means that the concept of 'subjectivity' is a central tenet of all forms of phenomenological understanding and enquiry. Subjectivity must be understood in terms of individual experience and contextual factors. However, individual experience must also be understood in the context of mankind as a social being and not in terms of isolated experience. Therefore subjectivity or individual experience does not occur in isolation. This implies the existence of 'intersubjectivity' which presumes that an individual is capable of both sharing experiences and understanding others' experiences, making sense of them and possibly integrating them with their own.

Lived experience/life-world

One of the main reasons why phenomenology and phenomenological research has evolved as a popular and widely used approach within health-related fields of inquiry is the fact that it is seen by many as the antithesis of positivist traditions that are associated with objectivity, a medical model of care and professional dominance. Another reason is the attraction of its holistic ethos, frequently associated with the term 'lived–experience'. Lived experience is attractive because it has connotations of real life as opposed to the contrived environments frequently associated with experimental research in laboratory environments.

Lived experience, in a phenomenological sense, is a more complex concept than it may appear on initial reading. 'Lived experience' is a translation from the original German word, 'lebenswelt'. 'Life-world' of lived experience is a more accurate translation of this term. 'Lebenswelt' is associated with the world of immediate experiences and one that is not contaminated by theoretical explanations or reflexivity. In other words it is the 'natural' world which is pre-theoretical and naïve, in the sense that it is uncomplicated by other factors. This concept of 'natural world' is central to phenomenological thinking and research and this centrality means that the role of the phenomenological researcher is not scientific analysis, but rather discovering the essence of meaning of everyday experiences (Colaizzi, 1978).

TRADITIONS WITHIN PHENOMENOLOGY

There has been a tendency to consider phenomenology and research based on phenomenological approaches within two fairly distinct traditions. One could argue that this is somewhat ironic as the division of phenomenology in such a manner can also be seen as reductionist. Despite this irony, many researchers base their approaches on the epistemological and ontological assumptions evident in the work of Husserl (interpretivist) on the one hand or Heidegger and Gadamer (constructivist) on the other. These 'divisions' are frequently described as the distinctions between constructivist and interpretivist approaches. Some claim that the differences and similarities have been the subject of heated debate among philosophers and researchers at the expense of more relevant discourse on the value of phenomenology itself (Luft, 2005). Likewise, the terms interpretivist and constructivist have sometimes been used interchangeably, or at least the term interpretivist has been applied to Heideggerian phenomenology. For clarity, it should be noted that in the remainder of this section, the term interpretivism is used to describe Husserlian phenomenology and constructivism to describe Heideggerian perspectives.

Those who subscribe to an interpretative perspective believe that the social world cannot be fully understood, but they can explore and interpret it, albeit in an incomplete way. As indicated, Heidegger differed from Husserl in that he believed that meaning is always contextual. In other words, meaning is achieved in the context of something else and not in isolation. Meaning must be understood in terms of such factors as one's humanity, sociological factors or life situation among other things (Luft, 2005). The constructivist perspective therefore argues that all forms of social knowledge are constructed within contexts.

Interpretivism and constructivism also differ in terms of their understanding of the role of those who undertake research. Those who operate from an interpretivist perspective claim that their findings are based on an interpretation of reality, which is founded on a level of 'objectivity' achieved through a process referred to as 'bracketing'. Bracketing is one of the core terms associated with phenomenological traditions in research and one of the core distinctions between the interpretivist and constructivist traditions.

The interpretative tradition argues that researchers must and can 'bracket' issues relating to their own biases, previous experience or other factors that might potentially influence their interpretation of the respondents' reports of their reality or life-world. Conversely, constructivists argue that researchers are themselves part of the social world and that it is implausible if not impossible to set aside one's previous experiences. The researcher is seen as a collaborator in the construction of one's lived experiences. Likewise, the researcher is part of the real world and as such the methods of collating and reporting the data reflect a collaborative effort.

THE ROLE OF THE RESEARCHER IN PHENOMENOLOGICAL RESEARCH

Phenomenological research is based on the stories or narrative accounts of respondents. Such accounts are accessed through conversations or interviews, but data collection and analysis methods as well as the role of the researcher are somewhat different in interpretivist and constructivist approaches.

We have already referred to 'bracketing' and the distinctions between both main perspectives. Interpretivist-based research assumes that meanings of experiences are unique to the individual and that the function of the conversation or interview is to describe experience rather than ascribe external meaning to experiences. The central purpose of the conversation is to probe the phenomenon until the essence of the meaning is illuminated. In terms of process, the function of the conversation requires an inductive approach, where the data that emerges drives the interview process and is thus not predetermined. The researcher engages in an unstructured process and follows the data through close and attentive listening, aimed at arriving at a deep understanding of the phenomenon under consideration. The interview process, therefore, is non-directive in nature and based on one-to-one interviews on the understanding that individual experience is unique.

From a constructivist perspective the role of the researcher in data collection is understood to be somewhat different. As already said, the notion of 'bracketing' is not seen as being consistent with Heideggerian phenomenology. In fact the researcher is seen as being an important element of the experience. Researchers are understood as individuals who use their previous experience as a means of contributing to or arriving at a wider understanding of the essential meaning of phenomena. The interviewer is seen as having particular skills at uncovering and making explicit issues that are taken for granted as mundane or 'everyday'. Therefore, the researcher believes their function is to help explain or construct reality, based on interpretations already arrived at by individuals.

Within this perspective, it is also important that the conversation engaged in is based on the use of everyday language and takes the form of a dialogue between the researcher and the participant. As with all forms of phenomenological research, the use of the term 'participant' as opposed to 'subject' implies a partnership within a process as opposed to an unequal relationship in reductionist-based research. In-depth interviewing is the norm within this tradition. Another distinction between interpretivist and constructivist perspectives is that constructivist research allows for the use of both individual and group interviews as well as appreciating the potential value of observation or other means of data collection. Additionally, multiple interviews may be used.

DATA ANALYSIS

Analysis of data, as with other aspects of the research journey, differs between the traditions, but they share some common elements also. The researcher is seen as needing to have a deep understanding of the data. Researchers are required to immerse themselves in the data through ongoing exposure to tapes, transcripts or field notes so they can arrive at an in-depth understanding of the meaning of the phenomena. In order to do so a variety of analytical 'frameworks' has been described which are intended to assist the researcher in arriving at meaning through a system of 'checks' and 'balances'. These frameworks are intended to ensure the authenticity and trustworthiness of the data and its understanding or interpretation. The frameworks, such as that proposed by Colaizzi (1978), should not be confused with a reductionist approach. The intent of these frameworks is to guide the process, not seek causal or other relationships.

The frameworks generally propose some form of coding of data. In order to achieve relevant coding, the data is normally transcribed into written form. Initial coding may be refined and further interviews may be undertaken to help clarify meaning or arrive at a deeper understanding of the phenomena. This is normally the process that is engaged in, but as indicated earlier, the data guides the process of both data collection as well as data analysis.

11
Grounded Theory

Learning Outcomes:

On completion of this chapter the reader will be able to:

- discuss the principles of grounded theory
- explore differing perspectives of grounded-theory approaches
- understand the process of grounded-theory research
- debate the key considerations in choosing grounded theory in health-promotion research.

INTRODUCTION

The term 'grounded theory' was introduced by Glaser and Strauss in the 1960s. In this research approach the researcher does not set out with a particular theory or hypothesis to prove or disprove, rather the research begins with a research area or topic and allows the data that emerges to direct the focus of the research. One of the key distinguishing features of the grounded-theory approach is that the research itself is inductive in nature. Inductive approaches imply that the researcher has a central role in that they engage in a process of data collection and theory generation simultaneously so that theory emerges consistently throughout the research process. In that sense both the process and outcome of research is important. A key consideration for researchers in grounded-theory approaches is that the voices of participants can be heard through the data and are represented in an authentic manner.

Grounded theory can be understood as an attempt to close the gap between theory and research by grounding the theory in empirical data (Grix, 2004). Indeed Glaser and Strauss (1967:viii) themselves referred to grounded theory as 'closing the embarrassing gap between theory and empirical research'. Grounded theory is sometimes referred to as an approach, but is more commonly understood as a specific type of research design. A grounded-theory research design is thorough and time-consuming but it is well suited to health-promotion research. The attraction of grounded-theory approaches to this field of research relates to the fact that it not only endeavours to illuminate the experiences of others, but also seeks to generate theory specific to their experiences. Therefore grounded theory would, for example, be an apt approach to research which is concerned with the development and support of advocacy among marginalised groups. It is also particularly relevant in areas about which little is currently known.

GROUNDED THEORY – DIFFERING PERSPECTIVES

Glaser and Strauss (1967) developed the grounded-theory approach as a result of their commitment to practical research and their awareness of the need for theory that is grounded in the experience of people and their social processes. Glaser and Strauss acknowledged that the primary task of the researcher is to verify existing theory but they were further cognisant of existing phenomena which were not measurable and quantifiable within traditional research approaches. Thus they argued that researchers also needed to engage in the generation of theory that could be later tested within traditional approaches. They advocated grounded theory as a possible way to do this as the grounded-theory approach would allow researchers to illuminate new phenomena which could be later tested within traditional research approaches such as positivism or naturalistic inquiry.

As grounded theory continued to evolve some differing philosophical assumptions underpinning understandings of grounded theory began to emerge between Glaser and Strauss and we see the development of two approaches to grounded theory. 'Classic' or interpretivist grounded theory has become associated with Glaser while constructivist grounded theory has become associated with Strauss and Corbin. The divide occurred as a result of differing ontological positions. Glaser's approach to grounded theory incorporates an understanding of the researcher as separate and objectively looking in on the social processes engaged in, while Strauss and Corbin argue that the researcher, rather than objectively representing what they see, actually interprets and creates a theory of social processes influenced by their own understanding of the world (Strauss and Corbin, 1990). Glaserian emphasis in grounded theory is on social realism. This means that Glaser assumes the world is factual with shared meanings and that the researcher can come to know this through the process of data collection. Straussian emphasis is on constructivism. This means that the researcher constructs and shapes the theory from the data available to them and in providing the lenses with which to read the research they add further to the lucidity of the description. The nature of the differing perspectives points to the need for a researcher to adopt a grounded-theory approach to take account of their ontological position with regard to research before adopting a particular approach. In other words the researcher must have arrived at an understanding of how they perceive their role as a researcher. Do they perceive that they objectively represent the phenomena under investigation (classic) or are they actively engaged in interpretation of the phenomena (constructivist)? Therefore, in grounded theory it is important that the researcher is specific with regard to their ontological position.

GROUNDED THEORY – PROCESS

In grounded theory the researcher may be examining either a phenomenon or a general area of interest. They familiarise themselves with the reality being studied, otherwise known as 'the field', at a very early stage. However, the parameters are not tightly set as the data that emerges during the process leads the researcher into the next relevant area which may not have been considered initially. What is important in a grounded-theory approach is that the researcher has not set limits with regard to scope, population or research themes prior to engaging with data collection. It is the data itself that guides the researcher in developing the next stage of the research; thus the research design is emergent in nature and guided by the experience of the phenomena rather than by the researcher's agenda. The researcher may employ any data-collection technique that they perceive relevant in order to illuminate the area of interest to them. The consideration at this stage is with regard to the appropriateness of the research methods for the phenomena or population under investigation.

Once the data-collection process begins, coding of data and data analysis must begin simultaneously, as the results of the data analysis influence the decision the researcher makes with regard to the next avenue for the research. The researcher creates categories for each new section of data emerging. In collecting, coding and analysing the data simultaneously the researcher is engaging in what is termed the constant-comparison method. Thus the researcher continues to assign codes to new sections of emerging data until no new data or codes are emerging. Once this happens data saturation is considered to have occurred indicating to the researcher that the data-collection process is completed and a new phase of the research may begin; that of interrogating the codes and categories created in order to understand how they relate to each other. This process is termed theoretical sampling. The theoretical-sampling stage can be a lengthy one in which the researcher is immersed in their data and codes in order to discover their relationships to each other. During this phase the researcher writes many memos attempting to identify the connections between codes and categories. Once this process is completed the researcher may then begin the process of articulating the emerging hypotheses and theories that are grounded in the data. The researcher may find they need to make several attempts at this task before they arrive at a theory that they are confident represents their findings. Grounded-theory researchers often represent their theories in the form of models, as this is an effective way of visually presenting their emergent theory.

During the process of data analysis the researcher engages in reviewing relevant literatures. This is not done prior to data collection, rather the accessing of literatures happens simultaneously during the research process as the data directs the researcher to the relevant conceptual frameworks that need to be explored. Thus as the research design and theory are emergent so too is the researcher's approach to the literature they explore. Glaser (2005) indicates the importance of this emergent approach to the research as central to grounded theory.

SOME CONSIDERATIONS IN CHOOSING GROUNDED THEORY IN HEALTH-PROMOTION RESEARCH

Because of its interpretive nature grounded theory has much to offer health-promotion research particularly in areas where not much is known about particular phenomena. Grounded theory by its nature is concerned with representing the reality of social processes and situations and in this way is commensurate with the values underpinning health-promotion activity such as empowerment and advocacy. However, grounded theory is uniquely intensive and is particularly time-consuming. For novice researchers it may appear quite daunting and in such cases it is better to have support from critical friends or those familiar with grounded-research processes so as not to become overwhelmed by the use of constant comparison and theoretical sampling. Grounded theory is a rigorous approach to conducting research, a particular strength of which lies in the acknowledgment of data as culturally saturated. Grounded-theory researchers attempt to represent current situations as closely as possible. They are committed to supporting participants by enabling their voices to emerge clearly in the research. This process means that participants are given opportunities to articulate their experiences, which guides the reader to understand the phenomena from the participants' perspective. Grounded theory gives the researcher scope to understand how and why people relate in particular ways and indeed the motivations behind behaviours. In the realm of health promotion a research approach that gives insight into particular behaviour and its motivation is of significant importance.

12
Action Research

Learning Outcomes:

On completion of this chapter the reader will be able to:

- understand the principles of action research
- distinguish action research from other research approaches
- discuss the cycle of action research.

INTRODUCTION

Action research is increasingly recognised as having much to contribute to health and social care as it is a form of research that is committed to the improvement of professional practice. Critical theory emerged as a research approach because of the concerns among proponents of the Frankfurt School such as Habermas, Adorno and Marcuse that current research methodologies did not recognise the historical, cultural and social situatedness of researchers and also that current research did not prioritise the social change agenda.

McNiff (2002:34) identifies the development of critical theory as a 'systematic approach to offer both an oppositional response to dominating influences and emancipatory hope'. She further identifies that other research traditions have emerged from critical theory such as critical feminist research and liberation theology and she positions action research within this framework also. The strength of an action-research approach lies in the encouragement of professionals to incorporate research as part of their professional practice which has significant long-term effects for the professional and for the organisation or community with whom they work.

Action research encourages practitioners to critique their context as well as the problem or issue being researched in order to come to a deeper understanding of the factors that influence their decision-making with regard to their daily practice. In keeping with the prioritisation of empowerment as a core principle of health promotion, action research is not something that is imposed upon others, rather, democratic processes are central to the research design and process.

> Action research should not be seen as a recipe or technique for bringing about democracy, but rather as an embodiment of democratic principles in research, allowing participants to influence, if not determine, the conditions of their own lives and work, and collaboratively to develop critiques of social conditions which sustain dependence, inequality or exploitation.
>
> (Carr and Kemmis 1986:164)

WHAT IS ACTION RESEARCH?

'Action research is simply a form of self-reflective inquiry undertaken by participants in social situations' (Carr and Kemmis, 1986:162). It has it roots in the work of Kurt Lewin (1946, 1958), who proposed that action research 'proceeds in a spiral of steps which is composed of a circle of planning, action and fact finding about the result of the action' (Lewin, 1946:38). This was further developed by Kemmis and McTaggart (1982) and Elliott (1991) into a series of cycles in which the practitioner/researcher observes, plans, acts, reflects and draws up a revised plan. We propose that, rather than understanding action research in terms of a simplistic cycle, a model of process is more appropriate.

Figure 12.1 Model of action research

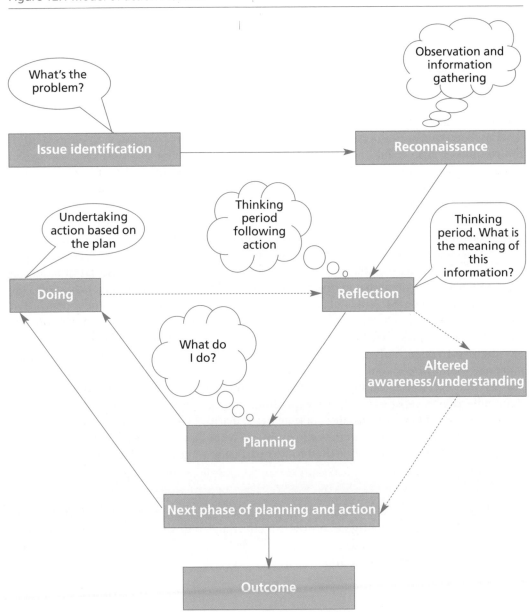

There is a danger of oversimplification in accepting the cycles as a given according to Winter and Munn-Giddings (2001). They point to the fluid nature of the reflection in that our concerns may shift as we become more aware of the political and cultural contexts that we work within. They also indicate that the emphasis on repeated cycles may give the impression that action research may take a long time to complete and may be difficult to sustain in work settings. However, this is not the case and action research can take place over a relatively short period of time; weeks and months, rather than years. Fostering an action-research culture within practice means that practitioners can interrogate (look critically at) their decisions and practice in order to move towards better or even best practice.

Thus action research need not be seen as an interruption to work but rather a way of furthering and developing the work already engaged in (Winter and Munn-Giddings, 2001:12). Practitioner research is an important link in closing the theory–practice gap and health-promotion practitioners can benefit from systematic reflection on their practice and research as a core component of this. Lawrence Stenhouse (1975), in his work with teachers, advocated the 'teacher as researcher'; that teachers were best positioned to carry out research with regard to their current practice and that those in higher education institutions were best positioned to support them in doing this research. The same can be said for health practitioners as they are best positioned to contribute to the development of theory in their professional area.

Action research differs from other forms of research in that not only does it offer descriptions of practice but the focus goes much deeper than these descriptions and provides explanatory farmeworks also. The focus is on understanding why the current situation is as it is and to engage in action in order to make changes to the situation. It is important that the practitioner/researcher make public the learning from the process (in some form, for example publishing an article in a journal or disseminating research at conferences) in order to support other practitioners who may gain insight from reading about the experiences of others.

Action research, unlike other forms of research, is practitioner-based and is conducted by practitioners who regard themselves as researchers also. It is responsive to social situations, it is intentionally political in that taking action is essentially a political act and it emphasises the value-base of practice (McNiff et al., 2003). Its key strength is in the generation of theory that is grounded in the practitioner's own practice and supported by the relevant published conceptual frameworks. We have argued elsewhere in this text that the polarising of research paradigms into quantitative and qualitative is overly simplistic and that these terms reflect more the means of data collection. Action research is an example of where this assertion applies. Action research can incorporate quantitative (such as questionnaire) and qualitative data-collection methods. Qualitative methods may include interviews, focus groups, document and content analysis, discourse analysis, diaries as well as other forms of data that may support a claim to have improved practice. The design is not prescriptive, rather it is motivated by the most relevant method for the particular stage of the research.

WHERE TO BEGIN?

Action research begins with an identification of the problem, issue or concern that the practitioner wishes to investigate in order to effect a change or improvement. Whitehead (1993) outlines a series of questions that are an effective way of ordering one's thinking with regard to action research. These are:

- What is my concern?
- Why am I concerned?

- What can I do?
- How can I show (evidence) that I am making an improvement?
- How can I judge (validate) that my conclusions are accurate?

Whitehead (1989) proposes a particular kind of question in the generation of what he terms 'living theory' in which the practitioner asks questions of the kind 'How do I improve my practice?'. Thus the improvement of professional practice is central to the action-research process.

Action research can be understood as involving a spiral of cycles of reflection and action. Within each cycle is a period of observation which then influences the planning of a particular action. This is followed by the implementation of the action, which is then reflected upon, and its impact is evaluated.

OBSERVATION

During the initial observation or reconnaissance phase the practitioner/researcher spends time diagnosing what the issues for consideration are. It involves a process of exploring the culture and context of the work they are engaged in. It involves deepening their understanding of why the issue is of particular concern to them and what are the factors that influence this situation. It is important at this stage and indeed throughout the research process that the researcher is also involved in the exploration of relevant published literatures and conceptual frameworks that will help to illuminate this understanding. For example, if the concern is with regard to a change process it is imperative that the researcher examine the conceptual frameworks that are widely published in this area. This serves to inform the researcher and also to ensure that the research is grounded in widely tested theory. The researcher may find as a result of their research that this theory does not fit their findings and may thus reject it in favour of their own theory which they have generated from their practice; however, this is done from an informed perspective. It is also important at this stage that the researcher, in collaboration with others, engage in this observation. It may be with a critical friend who is also a colleague, so that they may test their observations with others who may be able to offer formative critique.

PLANNING

Planning of action follows when the context and purpose of the project have become clear (Coughlan and Brannick, 2005). This incorporates planning what the action will look like in practice, but also attention to questions such as:
- How do I involve others collaboratively?
- What types of assurances and guarantees do I need to give to colleagues with regard to my research?
- What impact will the action have?
- What kind of data will I need to show that I have implemented the action?
- How will I gather the data?
- How will I validate the data that I have gathered so that it constitutes evidence of my claim to being successful?

ACTION

Once careful attention to planning has been given, the action can be implemented. It is important at this stage to pay careful and rigorous attention to data collection on the impact of the action.

REFLECTION

The period following action is spent in reflection and evaluation of the impact of the action. This may mean a re-examination of the initial observations and of the literatures studied as well as careful consideration of any data collected. As a result of the reflection and analysis the researcher may feel the need to alter the action and thus recommences the process of observation, planning and reflection in the second cycle or phase of the research.

DATA COLLECTION

As previously stated, action research may incorporate a variety of data-collection techniques and sources. Action researchers may employ a combination of techniques such as questionnaires, interviews, focus groups, diary keeping (by the researcher and other participants if appropriate). Data may also be obtained via letters, e-mail communications and telephone conversations. However, it is important to note that the researcher needs to ask permission to use the communication from the other person and also to ask them to validate the data piece by reading and agreeing that it is accurate. For example, the other person could sign and date the data piece in order to validate it. If the research is focusing on the improvement of a service, for example a cardiac rehabilitation unit, a brief questionnaire that clients can complete can aid the researcher in evidencing the improvement they claim. In the case of attempting to increase access to a service the increase in numbers as a result of some initiative may also serve as data. Such data pieces can serve as support to the other data-collection techniques being employed.

CRITICAL FRIENDS/COLLEAGUES

McNiff et al. (2003) identify the strengths of having a colleague as a critical friend as they can act as confidant and mentor and as they know the context well they can also offer support with regard to the micropolitics of work. It is important to pay attention to the choosing of a critical friend who can offer honest and formative critique, which can be difficult to do, but is very important in preserving the veracity of the research. Critical friends may also be involved in the validation of data.

VALIDATION

Validation refers to the truthfulness of the claim to knowledge made (McNiff et al., 2003). In action research the researcher must interrogate their process to test its validity, which can be explored using questions such as 'how can I show that my claim is true?'. Otherwise who is to say that the research report is not merely the researcher's own opinion? One way of addressing validation is to work with some critical friends or colleagues. In making the data available to them and in interrogating together the claims to knowledge that are being made with regard to the improvement of practice, colleagues may be able to offer critique as to whether the data supports this claim or not.

Being able to evidence a rigorous and systematic research approach also supports the validation process. In service provision it is possible that managers may be able to support the claims of practice improvement as a result of the action-research process, thereby offering validation. Making action-research accounts public, (e.g. discussing the research at staff meetings and practitioner forums, publishing on the internet and in relevant academic journals, presenting papers at conferences) further assists the validation process. Stenhouse (1985:17) strongly advocated the need to make action research public in the same way as is done with other forms of research as it is key to continuing the critique and refinement of knowledge.

GENERALISING FROM ACTION RESEARCH

Action research is often critiqued heavily for its local focus and lack of generalisability in the traditional sense. However, to understand the nature of action research it is important to examine the assumptions that underpin such critique. Action research tends to prioritise the empowerment of participants and to represent the data in terms of personal experiences in order to give voice to those who may otherwise be silenced. While action research may not be generalisable in the traditional sense of adhering to criteria such as random sampling of participants (not feasible if the practitioner is researching their own practice), the rigour and validation practices employed in action research ensure the legitimacy of the research. Indeed action research 'prides itself on producing specific practical changes and empowerment effects, at least as much as on any generalised findings' (Winter and Munn-Giddings, 2001:155).

ETHICS

The importance of and attention to ethics in action research is no less important or rigorous than in other forms of research (for a discussion on ethical principles see Chapter 14). However, some general principles to take note of are the voluntary participation of colleagues who are free to withdraw from the work at any stage without prejudice. Careful treatment of data is important so that participants are protected at all times, most specially if they are sharing data with a colleague and are working in the same organisation. Transparency in the research process and strict adherence to the avoidance of covert behaviours or research is also important. It is suggested that the researcher have an ethical statement that includes principles and procedures, which is made freely available to all concerned with the research. It helps allay any concerns and/or fears colleagues may have.

CONCLUSION

Action research is still considered controversial in some circles. In a society where technical rationalism is still the dominant form of knowledge prioritised in third-level education and where experts are those who make the decisions in the field of health and education, a form of research that positions the practitioner as one who also knows and who can also be a generator of knowledge is regularly resisted. Action research is a shift away from the hierarchical structures surrounding knowledge-generation towards a more democratically driven process. Given the consistent drive in health towards best practice and evidence-based practice, action research offers a unique opportunity to support practitioners in developing their skills in research and in ensuring that their practice is constantly informed by recent research and evidence. 'Good practice in action research is about justifiable decision making in situations involving human well being' (Winter and Munn-Giddings, 2001). The appropriateness of such a research process in the field of health and health promotion is evident.

13
Evaluation

Learning Outcomes:

On completion of this chapter the reader will be able to:

* define and distinguish between different types of evaluation
* discuss the reasons for undertaking an evaluation
* debate the key issues to be considered when planning an evaluation.

INTRODUCTION

Evaluation concerns assessment of the extent to which an action achieves a valued outcome (Nutbeam, 1998). In addition, there is usually a value placed on the process by which outcomes are achieved (Nutbeam, 1998). In other words evaluation is the process of assessing what has been achieved (outcome) and how it has been achieved (process). The Ottawa Charter's definition of health promotion outlined earlier identifies both valued outcomes and processes as central to health-promotion practice (WHO, 1986).

With the current emphasis on evidenced-based practice in healthcare it is not surprising that evaluation has become an integral component of health-promotion programmes and interventions. The extent of the evaluation will depend very much on the reason for the evaluation and the expertise and funding available. Evaluations can be carried out internally or by an external evaluator. External evaluation may be opted for in order to limit bias in the process. To ensure accuracy in evaluation it is best built into a programme at the planning stage rather than added on at a later phase when the opportunity to collect baseline data is no longer an option.

It is vital to decide at the planning stage the outcome criteria on which the efficacy of the programme will be evaluated. Failure to agree with key stakeholders what will be considered successful outcomes can lead to conflict and unrealistic expectations. For example those involved in running a return-to-work programme for women in disadvantaged communities may consider a programme successful when the participant's self-worth and confidence are sufficiently increased for her to consider applying for a job. An outside agency, on the other hand, may only consider the programme successful if a high proportion of the participants are in gainful employment at the end of the programme.

Evaluation in health promotion is performed for a variety of reasons:

* to establish the effectiveness of different health-promotion models, methods and strategies in order to inform future decisions, plans or policy
* to provide an evidence base for an intervention so that individuals and communities are offered programmes that can achieve the best possible outcomes
* to prevent reinvention of the wheel by informing other health promoters of the effectiveness or indeed problems associated with different methods and strategies

- to ensure cost-effectiveness and quality of health-promotion programmes
- to secure ongoing funding by justifying resource use and allocation.

TYPES OF EVALUATION

There are three forms of evaluation to consider when appraising the success of a programme: formative evaluation, process evaluation and outcome or summative evaluation.

1. **Formative evaluation** is conducted prior to the implementation of a programme. The data collected during this stage is used to inform the design of the programme. Meyer and Dearing (1996:46) define formative evaluation as 'the systematic incorporation of feedback about one or more components of a planned activity before communication with a target audience'. This feedback can be obtained either before or after the programme is created. This type of evaluation helps to identify and rectify potential inadequacies in the programme design and can be used to validate the needs assessment. While formative evaluation adds time and financial costs to preparing a programme, it is time well spent. However, it must be stressed that it will not guarantee programme success. Data-collection processes may include interviews, focus groups and surveys. Feedback on the programme design may be obtained by carrying out a pilot study or alternatively by inviting critique from colleagues or experts in the field.

2. **Process evaluation** takes place at various stages during the implementation of a programme. It involves evaluating what went on during the process of implementing the programme. The advantage of this type of evaluation is that you can establish whether the programme was carried out according to the plan. This provides an opportunity to rectify any aspects that may not have been implemented as planned. Alternatively the programme may have been implemented to plan but may not be proceeding as expected. Evaluation that pays attention to the implementation stages can support the practitioner in dealing with any unforeseen circumstances. The process can be evaluated by a combination of feedback from programme participants and trusted colleagues, observation and self-assessment using reflective practice (the process of critically reflecting on one's own practice). The importance of client participation was brought to the fore by the World Health Organization (1978) claim that 'people have the right and duty to participate individually and collectively in the planning and implementation of their health care'. Therefore it is important to get feedback from participants. This can be obtained from focus groups, comment sheets or suggestion boxes, or another useful method is to ask participants to anonymously record on comment cards up to five suggestions on areas for improvement and to submit ideas as to how these could be achieved. These ideas can then be considered for incorporation into current and future programmes. Feedback should be sought on any other issues relating to the programme, for example the room layout, the suitability of the venue and appropriateness of materials to the target audience. Practitioners may also want to know if the material was presented in a way that was easy to understand and appropriate and acceptable to the participants.

Feedback from colleagues or co-facilitators of a programme can also be invaluable; however, this must be given in an honest and respectful manner. Critical reflection is also a useful evaluation tool. Some questions that the practitioners may ask themselves to facilitate their reflections are:
- Did the session or programme run according to plan?

- If not, why not?
- What did I do well?
- What might I do differently if I was to run this session or programme in future?

Some practitioners choose to adopt an action-research approach as part of their evaluation. It serves as a useful way to structure their critical reflections on their own practice.

3. Outcome or summative evaluation usually happens at the end of a programme or at the completion of various stages of a phased programme. The purpose of outcome evaluation is to ascertain the effects of the campaign or programme on the target audience. In other words were the objectives of the programme achieved? It is impossible to answer this question without completing an outcome assessment.

There are various methods of conducting an outcome evaluation. The specific programme needs and the resources available largely determine the method selected. At the end of a six-week assertiveness programme, for example, participants may be invited to complete an assertiveness inventory. They may also be asked to identify how their behaviour has changed since partaking in the assertiveness group and how they perceive the programme will impact on their future behaviour. This is referred to as a *post-test-only* design, as data is collected from the programme participants on completion of the programme and not prior to or during the process. While it is relatively easy and cost-effective to ascertain this type of information, its validity is questionable. The practitioners cannot evidence what has changed as they have no baseline data to measure against, therefore they cannot be sure that it is participation in the programme alone that has brought about any change.

Outcome evaluation could also be achieved by comparing pre-and post-intervention measures. In a *pre-test/post-test* design data is collected prior to an intervention and the measures are repeated using the same instruments following the intervention. This model is useful to determine if a change in knowledge, attitude or behaviour has occurred. While a pre-test/post-test design is certainly an improvement on the post-test-only design it cannot claim with certainty that the change was directly brought about by the health promotion intervention. It is possible that the participants were exposed to other information or life events that impacted on or resulted in the change in knowledge, attitude or behaviour. Therefore care is needed with regard to claims that can be substantiated in the evaluation process.

Adding a control group to the pre-test/post-test design provides a third type of outcome evaluation referred to as *pre-test/post-test with control group* design. As with the pre-test/post-test design, data is collected before and after the intervention. The difference here is that data is collected from a control group as well as the intervention group. In this design participants are randomly assigned to either the intervention group or the control group. The idea here is that any pre-intervention differences in the participants should be evenly distributed in each group. Thus the outcome should result solely from the intervention. However, it is essential to ensure that contamination of conditions does not occur. For example, if practitioners teach the intervention group a specific skill you must ensure that participants do not communicate this skill to the control group. This is best achieved by allowing no communication between the intervention and control groups for the period under study.

PLANNING AN EVALUATION

A number of key issues to be considered when planning an evaluation are listed below:

> What is the purpose of evaluation?
> What resources are required?
> What will be the focus of the evaluation?
> What evaluation design will be used?
> Who will be involved in the evaluation process?
> Who will carry out the evaluation?
> Who will have access to the results of the evaluation?

The following guide is to assist the reader in deciding the type of evaluation to incorporate into the programme at the planning stage.

What is the purpose of the evaluation?

If the programme is evidence-based and the purpose of the evaluation is to improve one's own practice as a health promoter, one may decide that feedback from participants and self-evaluation are appropriate. On the other hand if the purpose of the evaluation is to secure funding or to establish effectiveness, more systematic and formal procedures are required.

What resources are necessary and available for evaluation?

Powell (1999) advises that knowledge, skills and administrative support are required when performing an evaluation. Without such supports it is difficult to effectively engage in evaluation. A number of barriers to evaluation exist in health-promotion practice. The cost of evaluation in terms of time, personnel and finance must be considered. The planning must take into account whether the cost of the evaluation comes from the programme budget or is to be funded separately. A large-scale evaluation of a community programme may be costly in terms of time and resources. Therefore evaluators need to be aware of the timeframe available for completion of the programme and its evaluation. This may vary from a few months to a few years depending on the scale of the programme. The timing of the evaluation is also important. Stress levels measured at the end of a six-week stress-management programme may differ from those recorded three months later when the client has had an opportunity to incorporate the required changes into their lifestyle. However, if the evaluation process waits for six months the client may have incorporated other stress-management strategies and advice, which may influence the outcome.

What will be the focus of the evaluation?

The evaluator must decide whether the evaluation will focus on the outcome or the process. It is preferable to evaluate both. Due to limitations on resources and taking due consideration for the participants it is not always possible to evaluate everything about an intervention so it may be necessary to prioritise key outcomes. Thus the key outcomes prioritised must be closely related to the aims and objectives of the programme, so that the focus of the evaluation is to identify if the programme achieved what it set out to do.

What evaluation design will be used?

The type of data a practitioner wishes to collect determines whether the design is qualitative or quantitative. If numerical data is required such as scores and comparisons, a quantitative design that incorporates a control or comparison group may be used. Alternatively if the evaluator wishes to incorporate the voices of the participants, a qualitative design of interviews and focus groups may be more appropriate. If the aim of an intervention is to bring about a change in behaviour, observation or recording would be appropriate. On the other hand if the objective was to bring about a change in knowledge a questionnaire might be more suitable. Sometimes a combination of qualitative and quantitative methods such as questionnaires and interviews is used to triangulate findings. Combining methods can help address the limitations of using a single methodology. Whatever method of data collection is selected it is vital that the data is reliable, valid, unbiased and culturally appropriate (McKenzie and Smeltzer, 2001).

It is also important that the evaluation is conducted in an ethical manner. This includes such issues as protecting the welfare of all participants and presenting findings accurately and in a balanced manner.

Who will be involved in the process?

When collecting data the evaluator must decide if input is required from all or just some of the key stakeholders. In order to be able to justify conclusions drawn from an evaluation it is useful to collect data from a variety of stakeholders such as programme participants, the wider community and the health-promotion agencies. Ideally the voices of all of those who have participated in or are affected by the programme should be heard. If the target audience is large, then a sample may be selected using probability or non-probability sampling. Sampling should be guided by clear and well-established research principles and procedures. Thus evaluation needs to be carried out by those *au fait* with research.

Who will carry out the evaluation?

It must be decided whose responsibility it is to evaluate the programme. Evaluation may be completed by the design team, the health-promotion practitioner delivering the programme or by an external evaluator. Insider evaluation (conducted by those delivering the programme) is more cost-effective and has the added advantage that the person is knowledgeable of the background to the project. On the other hand it could be argued that an outside evaluator may have more research expertise and may bring a fresh perspective and an unbiased attitude to the process. The motivations behind the evaluation and the plans with regard to dissemination of findings often dictate who is best positioned to conduct the evaluation. If the results are to be used 'in-house' then insider evaluation is adequate; however, if the results are to be used to source funding or to demonstrate accountability, an unbiased external evaluator may be called for.

Who will have access to the results of the evaluation?

The depth and detail included in an evaluation report will be influenced by who will have access to the results. Whether the evaluation is to be published or not is a key consideration for the style of report that will be produced. Once an evaluation is conducted it is important that the research is disseminated to user groups, practitioners and policy makers in the health-promotion field. This ensures widespread implementation of effective programmes, and curtailment of the implementation of less effective programmes (King, Hawe and Wise,

1998). There is some concern in health-promotion circles that the full potential of health-promotion programmes is not being achieved because of insufficient transfer of new knowledge about effective programmes from research into practice (Johnson *et al.*, 1996) resulting in continuous reinvention of the wheel. Therefore dissemination of evaluation research is central to the improvement of health-promotion practice.

14
Ethics and Health-promotion Research

Learning Outcomes:

On completion of this chapter the reader will be able to:
- understand the ethical principles associated with research
- debate the application of ethical practice in research.

INTRODUCTION

Any discourse with regard to health-promotion research should make reference to ethics. While it is the case that ethical considerations have traditionally been associated more with research involving invasive procedures or clinical trials, there is an increasing recognition that the principles of ethical research should underpin all research.

The history of research is not a universally proud one in terms of ethics and this was perhaps most obvious with experiments on humans during the period of the Third Reich, although concern is not exclusive to this historical period. The Nuremberg Code of Ethics, which was formulated following the Second World War, was perhaps the most notable international effort to set out a universal charter or code of conduct to guide research practice. However, despite this development and the subsequent adoption of ethical standards, codes of practice and conduct by most healthcare professionals, there have been instances where unethical practice and research have occurred. While any code of conduct such as this should protect the public in the first instance, it should have the simultaneous effect of protecting the reputation of research practice.

ETHICS AS A FORM OF PROTECTION

When examples of unethical research are given, one thing becomes obvious very quickly. Those who were subjected to unethical research were in an unbalanced power arrangement and many if not all could be described as vulnerable. In the case of the Nuremberg experiments, the subjects were prisoners. Caplan (1992), in a review of the infamous Tuskegee study in Alabama, pointed out that the subjects in that study were offered 'special' free treatment, but the subjects were all drawn from an African American population. Likewise in the case of the controversies relating to organ retention from babies in both the UK and Ireland in more recent years, the isssue of equity also needs consideration. Those parents or next of kin from whom *informed* consent should have been obtained were likely to be in a distraught state and even if or when consent forms were used, it is likely that they were not well understood. Therefore while procedures for 'form filling' may have been adhered to, the spirit as well as the letter of procedural compliance becomes an important ethical issue in its own right. It can also be argued that those who are 'patients' are invariably in an imbalanced power relationship, with the balance of power firmly resting with the health professional.

The essential reason for adherence to ethical standards is of course protection. Protection of the individual or group under investigation, protection of the individual researcher and of research as an area of practice. Decisions made in research practice relate to the making of moral choices and are interlinked with the personal beliefs and values of the researcher in the context of the cultural influences and norms in which the research is undertaken. The moral justification for undertaking particular research (or not) may be influenced by beliefs drawn from differing philosophical perspectives. *Utilitarian* philosophy might argue that the 'end justifies the means'. Those adhering to a *deontological* philosophy follow the belief that actions are either right or wrong in themselves and therefore all research actions are driven by motives which are universal and should be subject to universal 'laws' or rules of practice. Those who are driven by a philosophy of *relativism* might suggest that all standards must be viewed and understood in the context of the culture or environmental circumstances in which they occur.

While those engaged in or concerned with research are likely to debate these perspectives – and most likely will never arrive at a consensus! – it is also the case that there is general consensus on the fact that research participants and subjects must be protected and have rights. Naturally, as far as human beings are concerned, this requirement is even more important. Specifically LoBionda-Wood and Harber (1998:277) argue 'that human subjects have the right not to be harmed physically, psychologically or emotionally'.

As a protection, it is now common practice in academic and health and social service agencies, that all research projects involving human beings must achieve the approval of ethics committees before access to populations is agreed. Additionally it is becoming more common that respected professional or research-based journals require authors to provide evidence of ethical clearance prior to consideration of manuscripts for publication. At the very least, they will require evidence of compliance with ethical standards of practice. Beauchamp and Childress (2001) propose the following as the four main principles of ethical research in Western societies: beneficence, non-maleficence, respect for autonomy and justice.

Others, such as Parahoo (1997), argue that other principles such as fidelity, justice, veracity and confidentiality are also ones that underpin research. An increasing volume of research is being undertaken on health-related matters among both clinical and non-clinical populations (Grinyer, 2001). While ethical requirements in research practice involving clinical research are well established, it is important that research with non-clinical populations is guided by equally high standards of ethical practice. This should apply to everyone involved in any aspect of research, either conducting, facilitating or utilising research findings (Eckstein, 1998).

Beneficence

This principle refers to the moral position of always 'doing good'. In relation to research, this principle means that researchers should be driven by an ethos or value of ensuring that the rights and welfare of subjects or participants are of paramount importance. In practice this means that the rights of participants must always supersede the requirements of research protocols, especially in situations where there might be conflicts. It also means that even in situations where participants provide consent to researchers for participation in a study and subsequently change their minds, the rights of participants must not merely be acknowledged, but actively defended.

Non-maleficence

Non-maleficence refers to the notion of 'doing no harm'. It is firmly rooted in the principles espoused by Hippocrates and is probably the oldest ethical principle associated with health-service provision. Indeed, it is easier to cite examples of how this principle might be applied from clinical medicine than from research. While it might seem that this principle of research is somewhat redundant if research practice operates on principles of beneficence, it needs to be pointed out that being driven by the principle of always doing good does not invariably mean that that no harm will result from our actions. One of the key issues related to this principle is the combined issue of intent and risk. It is generally considered unethical to undertake research that is known to result in harm to an individual. While some may argue that the eventual outcome of such research may be for the greater good, this argument is generally not acceptable. It is also possible that any intervention or research may possibly result in some harm, but it is vital that the intent to harm is not present and that adequate measures are taken to ensure that any possible risk is minimised or removed. Associated with the notion of intent is the requirement under this principle that participants be protected from harm. We should of course remember that in some situations actions may have more than one effect, classically one good effect and one undesirable outcome. This is referred to as the *principle of double effect*. In such situations it is mainly the intent of the actions that requires ethical consideration. In the first instance the action undertaken should itself be judged in the context of that action being itself intrinsically good – or at least neutral.

If the action meets those criteria, then the issue of intent becomes paramount. In all cases, it must be the clear intention that the positive effect is the one intended, despite the fact that it is known that there is a distinct possibility of a simultaneous negative effect. When consideration is given to the action being engaged in, the potential negative effect should be less than the positive effect intended.

Perhaps it might be useful to provide some examples. In clinical-practice situations one of the classic examples of double effect relates to the removal of a malignant growth in a womb during pregnancy. In that regard, the clear intent is life-saving even though there may be a predictable risk to the foetus. Clearly, on a broader front, when a surgeon engages in a life-saving operation, harm will inevitably be done to tissues, bones or organs not directly associated with the site of surgery, which will be damaged in gaining access to or repairing a site.

In research settings, application of this principle is sometimes practically challenging, for example during drug trials, patients are put at risk. Precise risks may be unknown, but what is known is that potential risks are involved, even though the clear intent is to develop drugs that will improve health. However, despite the challenging nature of this ethical principle, it is absolutely vital that it is upheld and is seen to be upheld.

Respect for autonomy

This principle is also sometimes referred to as the principle of respect for persons. This is an interesting distinction but in effect shows that there is a complex understanding of the interplay between autonomy and individuality. Gillon (1986) argues that autonomy refers to the capacity of an individual to think, decide and then act freely and unhindered based on that thought and decision. This definition has clear implications for researchers in terms of the respect for autonomy. Firstly, respect must be clearly shown for the beliefs, values, thoughts, decisions and actions of individuals. However, autonomy is also linked with the concept of capacity. It clearly obliges researchers or practitioners to respect the right to self-determination and individuality. However, researchers must take due cognisance of individuals' capacity to be autonomous and support that, or in cases where there is limited capacity, to ensure adequate protection is provided.

In research, this is one of the reasons why the notion of *informed* consent as opposed to just consent is extremely important. It is vital that informed consent forms an explicit element of research involving human beings. Likewise, in all research where individuals may have limited capacity or are vulnerable, researchers who uphold the principle of respect for autonomy will put in place adequate and appropriate supports or protection for such persons to ensure their rights to individuality or self-determination are upheld.

Justice

The principle of justice can also be described as 'fairness'. Fairness and justice relate to more than simply fair treatment during research. This principle applies to selection of participants, the research process and indeed outcomes. In relation to selection of participants, the principle of justice dictates that there should be equity in terms of selection. In terms of the protection of human beings it particularly refers to the protection of vulnerable populations. It means that coercion should not be used and that issues of 'positional authority' need to be considered in the selection process. Potential participants must be afforded proper protection from undue influence to agree to take part in research. This is the case in particular with individuals in prison, in institutions or persons with limited intellectual or cognitive capacity. However, the principle of justice applies to the fair and equitable treatment of individuals, once they are actually involved as research participants. Likewise, following completion of research, they should also be afforded access to the research findings.

Parahoo (1997) argues that ethical principles can be considered in terms of four principle *rights*, namely the right to full disclosure; the right to self-determination; the right to non-maleficence and the right to privacy, anonymity and confidentiality.

ENSURING THE RIGHTS OF HUMAN RESEARCH PARTICIPANTS

While it is not possible to deal both succinctly and comprehensively with each of these principles and rights simultaneously, it may be useful to provide some guidance on the application of these principles. While issues are presented under distinct headings there are some areas of overlap. The primary consideration in research is the dignity of the human being (Polit and Hungler, 1995). Inherent in this consideration are a number of rights. In our view, these include the right to respect, the right to self-determination, the right to disclosure, the right to refuse participation, the right to fair treatment and the right to privacy, confidentiality and anonymity.

The right to respect

When planning and undertaking any form of research, it is vital that the dignity and integrity of all participants is respected. Upholding this right should guide all research practice with human beings, irrespective of the research approach. Respect for human beings means that human life has intrinsic value in its own right and that individuals need to be treated with respect based on their achievements and value (Harris, 1966). However, the emphasis on achievement and value may be somewhat problematic in that it suggests that there may be comparative value where human life is concerned. Others reject this concept of potential comparative value and there is widespread consensus that all individuals should be entitled to equal treatment and respect irrespective of achievement (Rumbold, 2000). This implies that in the context of research involving human beings, participation should not be viewed as a means to an end but rather all individuals must be treated equally.

It is vital that any information provided or data collected is only used for the purposes intended. Participants must have every opportunity to be assured that they know how the information will be used, and that they are aware of the scope of the research. From a researcher's perspective, it is important that they collect, collate, store and destroy data or information in a means consistent with both the letter and spirit of data-protection legislation.

Therefore, the researcher must ensure that participants:

- are normally in a position to make a free choice to participate in research
- can be assured of the right to withdraw consent at any time
- are treated fairly and protected from potential harm
- have their personal information dealt with in a private manner and are assured of confidentiality.

Choosing to participate in or withdraw from research freely

Frequently the issue of free choice is portrayed as informed decision making. However, consent must be provided on the basis of valid, relevant and full information. Firstly, the issue of disclosure of information by the researcher needs to be considered. It is important that as much information as possible is made available to participants.

For consent to be informed, the researcher must consider the issue of *competence*. Not alone must information be available to participants, but researchers must be confident that participants are competent to make voluntary choices and possess full information which they comprehend (Nachmias and Frankfort-Nachmias, 1992). Effectively, this means that in all situations it is important that information is made available in a means that participants can understand. Where participants have special needs, such as impaired vision, then information may be given verbally or through Braille. The language used should take cognisance of the level of participants' literacy skills and their ability to understand technical terms. If there is a possibility that participants have difficulty with authority figures, then a researcher should ensure that an independent advocate or 'friend' of the participant's choice can attend information sessions prior to a decision to participate.

The issue of power relationships needs to be considered. Many researchers do not consider themselves to be in positions of power or influence when conducting their research, but participants might perceive them to be. The important issue when considering a sample or participants is the issue of autonomy and free choice from the perspective of the participants.

When conducting research the researcher must be aware of power or perceptual differentials and the potential impact on the research process and therefore must do everything possible to negate such effects.

Fair treatment and protection from harm

Fair treatment commences at the design stage of research and should permeate every phase of the research process. Fair treatment means that selection of participants must be non-discriminatory irrespective of the nature of the data-collection methods or the sampling approaches. Fair treatment is important for the individual as well as for the research outcomes. For findings to either contribute to theoretical development or be generalisable as appropriate to the design, it is important that the selection process meets criteria that can provide evidence of fairness.

Principles of fairness and protection from harm should apply to those who agree to participate in research. However, these principles must also apply to those who choose not to participate. Those who choose not to participate in research or who withdraw at any stage must be protected from any immediate or longer-term negative consequences or discrimination. Indeed that is one of the main reasons why many advise against drawing samples from those with whom a researcher has any possible 'power' relationship.

Ensuring fair treatment is frequently facilitated through formal 'research contracts'. It is vital that contracts are both realistic and deliverable for all parties concerned and that any verbal or written contracts or 'understandings' with research participants are fully honoured.

Implicit in the notion of fair treatment is the avoidance of or protection of participants from harm. Within the context of health-promotion research it is unlikely that invasive procedures will be the norm, but much research in this field involves interviews or the disclosure of personal information. Researchers should always remember that disclosure of this nature may occasionally lead to upset and negative cognitive or emotional responses. There is a responsibility, therefore, on researchers to be available to participants for support or clarification. Additionally, researchers should put in place support structures that are available to any participant who becomes upset while participating in research projects or following such participation. Debriefing sessions are sometimes used and indeed autonomous counselling services are also sometimes arranged. While it might seem obvious, it is also important to emphasise the fact that any form of contact between a researcher and participants should be characterised by respect and dignity.

Privacy, confidentiality and anonymity

In an age of vastly expanding communication and means of sharing information the issues of privacy and confidentiality are important. These principles are addressed in the codes of conduct of virtually all professions for both practice and research. Both privacy and confidentiality are closely associated with the right to self-determination and as such the right to privacy and confidentiality of research participants is an extremely important issue where human beings are concerned. There are both ethical and pragmatic reasons for such an approach. In the first instance, the researcher is obliged to protect the individual, but equally (especially where sensitive topics are the subject of investigation) individuals may be either unlikely to participate or unwilling to divulge truthful answers if there is a possibility that their responses can be subsequently identified.

Within the context of the principle of self-determination, both privacy and confidentiality are associated with *control*. Privacy can be understood as individuals having control over the disclosure of information about themselves to others. This relates not only to the content of data being shared, but also to the means and circumstances of any disclosure. The right of individuals to disclose or withhold information about themselves through or following any research involvement must be respected. This includes the right to withdraw permission to disclose information.

Confidentiality refers to the management of shared information. In professional relationships and in research situations, trust is a factor of the context in which information (frequently of a sensitive and personal nature) is shared. In a research context, it is frequently the nature of the information itself that is important in contributing to knowledge formation or development. Therefore, the key issue becomes the protection of the identity of the individual informant or research participant and the conditions under which information will be used or made public. There is a clear expectation that information shared in trust will be used appropriately and that permission will be sought and granted to use such information. In order to avoid any potential conflict or misunderstanding, the importance of adequate and appropriate disclosure of the nature and purpose of the information-gathering and dissemination cannot be overstated. Indeed the procedures for the protection of participants' privacy and anonymity as well as the commitment to confidentiality should be explicit in the research contract or statement of consent. Guidelines for the appropriate storage of data should be explicitly stated in advance of the commencement of research. Participants should clearly understand who will have access to original data and how anonymity will be guaranteed in any publication of research.

15
Conducting Literature Reviews

Learning Outcomes:

On completion of this chapter the reader will be able to:

- appreciate the value of literature to research and practice
- recognise the hierarchies of evidence within literature
- discuss the process of reviewing literature.

INTRODUCTION

This chapter will examine the various sources of literature and the reasons for and process of evaluation of literature. In order that health-promotion practitioners can inform their practice with current research it is vital that they develop the skills to access relevant literature and information, judge the quality of that information, appraise the relevance of the information to their practice and identify the relative strengths and limitations of published literatures.

LITERATURE, WHAT IS IT AND HOW 'GOOD' IS IT?

The term 'literature' has a variety of meanings, but is traditionally associated with printed material or manuscripts, novels, periodicals, magazines, journals, newspapers and books. Increasingly literature is available electronically rather than necessarily in printed format. For the purposes of this text our references to 'literature' are specific to sources of published literature likely to inform professional and research activity in both the health and health-promotion fields.

WHY REVIEW LITERATURE?

Central to effective research is the ability to conduct a review of relevant literature. Within a research context, the term 'literature review' has gained a particular meaning, in so far as there is a normal expectation that relevant literature will have been critically appraised and presented in research proposals and presentation of findings. Part of the reason for this requirement is that sound evidence of the 'rationale' for undertaking research will be grounded in published literature. It is also important to situate research findings within published conceptual frameworks. Thus the researcher can see how the current research supports, adds to or even disagrees with the existing body of knowledge in the area under or proposed for investigation. A number of possible reasons for the inclusion of literature review in a research process are discovery/enquiry, learning/informing and building a case for the research.

WHERE TO START?

Accessing and reviewing literature may be undertaken simply because of a natural inquisitiveness relating to a topic. In other words, curiosity! Such curiosity can and will be satisfied through the discovery process of reviewing literature. Pragmatically, seeking evidence of what is already published on a topic area clearly assists a reader in discovering what information is already known and helps to avoid unnecessary repetition. This type of activity is essential to help inform clinicians, policy makers, health-promotion agents and the general public. This information, in turn, helps to influence decisions and actions as well as reactions. We have already referred to the evidence-based movement and the requirements to be able to 'defend' decisions on the basis of the most current information, trends or 'best practice'. Thus the issue of discovery or enquiry clearly becomes more than merely an idle curiosity.

From a professional perspective, reviewing current literature is imperative. Informing the professional practice of practitioners is central to the continuous evolution and improvement of professionalism. Keeping informed of the latest research through accessing literature is an effective way to do this. Reviewing literature involves a set of skills such as the adoption of a structured approach to the examination of a body of information, the sharing of that information either by the source with the individual reader or by dissemination from the reader to a wider audience, and engaging in critique of the efficacy and relevance of the arguments portrayed in the literature. From a research perspective, reviewing literature provides the reader with the opportunity to learn about a topic area as well as related issues. For example, the reader can learn who the leading scholars are in the field. They can discover the most current discourses. They can explore the research methods, approaches or practice guidelines most commonly used and thus develop a coherent defence of the reasons for particular approaches. Equally importantly, the literature can also inform the reader of core, evolving or divergent theoretical perspectives on health issues.

From a research perspective, it should be unnecessary to 'reinvent the wheel'. In other words, if research has definitively proved something, then it should not be necessary to do so again. This does not mean that existing knowledge cannot or should not be tested via replicated research. Indeed this is very often necessary in the process of creating standardised research instruments. But replication clearly requires a logical defence. From a research perspective, there is an expectation that researchers will present arguments that are coherent and comprehensive as well as compelling. Therefore, whether one is a novice researcher making a research proposal or an experienced researcher presenting findings from a study, there is an expectation that the researcher can present a good 'case' supporting their arguments. It is important that the sources of information (published literatures) used to support arguments are coherent, credible and as current as possible.

THE PROCESS OF REVIEWING LITERATURE

The process of reviewing literature involves the use of a structured approach to sourcing and appraising information. Anyone who has ever engaged in the process of searching literature will readily acknowledge the difficulty of setting both the scope and limits of the search; however, there are a number of approaches that can be taken.

Clearly, when undertaking a literature search, the search strategy will be informed by the individual's knowledge of the subject or topic area. For example, if the main purpose of the literature search is to discover broad information about a topic area, then background material may be sourced, so that the search strategy will be likely to draw on a wide range of sources and be more general in nature. However, if the researcher is seeking information on a specific aspect of a topic, then their search will be more refined and focused. In each of these situations, differing approaches and sources may be used.

Acknowledging these types of requirement, it is also necessary that literature searches are driven by curiosity; thus we would advise that the very simple questions of What? Who? Why? When? Where? and How? guide the search process. It is important for the researcher to discover issues such as:

• What research or information is available on a topic area or what aspects of the topic have already been addressed?
• What do I wish to do with the information I discover? This is particularly important in helping to identify relevant research questions.
• Who has previously undertaken research in this area? This would include who the target population has been, who has been excluded or included from previous studies.
• Who are the recognised 'experts' in the field?
• What are the likely sources of funding or support?
• Why was a particular research strategy or design utilised? Appropriateness of design is an important consideration in appraisal of findings.
• Why do I need or want information on this topic?
• When was the research undertaken? Currency of research findings or possibilities of change across time are important factors to be considered.
• Where has the research been carried out? It may also be useful to identify gaps where research has not been undertaken and why. It should not be assumed that research findings automatically transfer across settings or cultures.
• How does the process of the research undertaken influence the findings?

While these questions may appear overly simplistic, they address the essence of the enquiry needed to appraise research or the information being reviewed in terms of its utility, relevance or applicability.

As a general guideline, a search strategy should provide the researcher with a thorough and comprehensive coverage of the relevant topic area, enabling them to have sufficient resource material for their needs. This in turn points to the level of reading at different stages in the process. Initially, it is important to identify the sources of information and then plan an approach to sifting through the information itself. There is a wide range of potential sources, both primary and secondary. Primary sources normally refer to actual reports of studies undertaken or case studies, while secondary sources tend to include systematic reviews, meta-analyses, integrative reviews and research-based clinical guidelines. The most popular sources of literature are books, journals (including electronic databases), official reports, theses and conference proceedings.

There are strengths and limitations to each source. For example, official reports normally provide primary sources which are usually rich in detail. However, in many cases, reports are only published by the commissioning agency and have limited circulation or availability. Likewise, theses, particularly those at doctoral level, are normally extensive and rich in detail. However, they are often difficult to access, available for reading rather than on loan or only accessible on an inter-library loan basis. Theses have the strength of having been through a rigorous assessment process and benefit from the scrutiny of peers. Likewise some journals and professional magazines require articles to be reviewed by peers and experts in the particular field. This means that articles have been subject to a level of scrutiny that adds to their strength and quality. Articles in peer-reviewed journals such as these tend to be of a higher order than those which do not rely on primary research and are not peer-reviewed.

Irrespective of the source itself, finding the material will involve either a manual search through libraries or more commonly a search of electronic databases (or indeed a combination of both). It is worth noting that just as there is a variation between the quality of publications, there is also a difference between general and specialised libraries, in which the system of storing and cataloguing library stock may differ. Therefore it is important that anyone undertaking research becomes familiar with their own library as well as the resources available to them. Academic libraries generally provide the opportunity to search their catalogues and sometimes electronic databases through internet access. This is normally restricted to registered users, who in the main will be students of the institution. Increasingly in Ireland, this type of access is also being made available through health-service agencies, so that access to current information should be readily available for health-service employees. However, having access to and being able to search and review literature are not necessarily the same thing!

In relation to the catalogue of holdings of a library, it is important that you identify 'key words' or phrases associated with your topic area as soon as possible. These can then guide a general search of the literature within the holdings of the library. Use of the same 'key words' can guide an electronic search. This should generate initial resource material. It is important to keep track of the key words used and electronic databases searched, so that the scope of the search is evident in the written report.

EVALUATING RESEARCH-BASED LITERATURE

For anyone who has ever sought literature on a topic of interest the main problem is rarely related to finding literature. The sources of information have expanded exponentially with the advent of the internet and electronic databases and sources of information. The main problem is more commonly discerning what is of value and ranking the order of relevance of the information.

Once relevant literature has been found, it is necessary to evaluate the relative value of the information. Articles that have been peer-reviewed or have been subject to some form of expert review can normally be considered to be higher-order material than those that have not had that level of scrutiny in the publication process. However, it should not be automatically assumed that this is universally the case.

Pragmatically, it is also useful to access literature that has an abstract. Frequently, titles of articles may not fully reflect the content, so it is important as an initial filtering process to be able to form an initial judgment by drawing on the information in the abstract. This also helps to guide the reading, prioritise information and focus the direction of the review process.

Having focused the scope of the literature to be reviewed, perhaps the first issues a reader needs to be conscious of when reading literature are their own experience, beliefs and potential bias. Generally speaking, it is wise to read with an open mind and an inquisitiveness, rather than reading to attempt to prove one's own point or perspective. With topic areas where there is a plethora of information, it is also useful to access the most recent literature initially. This has the advantage of informing the reader of the most recent discourse in a particular field. It also provides the reader with useful signposts to earlier research or publications in the citations or bibliography section.

Following initial assessment of the medium (for example book or peer-review journal) in which the information is published, there are also several other levels of assessment that are important. It is important to remember the research focus and the level of the study in the overall 'hierarchy of evidence'.

When reading health-based research the reader must evaluate the merit and relevance of the study in the context of the methods used and the appropriateness of the design. Particular methodologies or research designs have traditionally been understood to be hierarchically organised in the medical field which has been hugely influential in health research. However it is equally important to recognise that hierarchies of evidence are more associated with the effectiveness of interventions than other forms of research. Therefore, the hierarchical position of evidence needs to be considered in terms of the type of research itself. While systematic reviews and randomised control trials (RCTs) are commonly cited as the highest level of evidence, these approaches also have limitations. RCTs are not appropriate for addressing many forms of research questions, nor may it always be possible or appropriate to undertake them. The strength of the evidence must be considered in terms of the appropriateness of the research approach for the topic under investigation.

While one can accept in general terms that hierarchies of evidence exist, these should be interpreted in the context of the types of study undertaken. It ultimately falls to the individual reader or researcher to arrive at an informed opinion on the quality and appropriateness of the evidence. In that regard there are a number of general questions or indicators that should be remembered and should guide that judgment, such as:

- Is the purpose of the study clearly stated?
- Is there, or should there be, a clear conceptual framework or theoretical perspective underpinning the study?
- Is there a logical 'fit' between the relevant sections of the published study?
- Is the literature considered appropriate within the context of the underpinning research paradigm?
- Is the design clearly articulated and are the methods used appropriate?
- Is the sampling procedure appropriate and clearly articulated?
- What, if anything, do the findings add to existing knowledge?
- What are the key strengths and limitations of the study?

16
Interviews

Learning Outcomes:

On completion of this chapter the reader will be able to:

- differentiate between an interview and a conversation
- distinguish between differing types of interview
- discuss the principles of effective interviewing.

INTRODUCTION

Interviews are a popular research tool in health-promotion research. They are useful particularly when the researcher wishes to explore the phenomenon under investigation in more depth. Interviews aid the researcher in understanding the meaning-making and significance that research participants place on circumstances. They are practical as they offer much flexibility and can be modified to fit various research situations (Punch, 1998). Interviews can yield a great deal of valuable information (Leedy and Ormond, 2005) and are thus a realistic and practical research tool to employ in a research design that is either qualitative in nature or that includes a qualitative component. Kvale (1996) identifies that an interview is in essence an interaction between two people on a topic of mutual interest and that it typifies the centrality of human interaction in the process of knowledge production. Cohen, Manion and Morrison (2000) argue that an assumption underpinning qualitative research is the social 'situatedness' of data. In other words that data is culturally saturated and that opinions articulated by participants in interview cannot be divorced from their socialisation and context. Therefore interviews, while they have the potential to generate culturally rich data, are also concerned with the generation of knowledge, which is created when two people actively engage in dialogue with each other. Thus interviews are inter-subjective as the process of the engagement means that they are neither completely objective nor subjective (*Ibid.*). The data itself cannot be treated as completely separate to the relationship between researcher and participant as both the data and the engagement is embedded within the research process.

DEFINING INTERVIEWS

An interview can be defined as a person-to-person interaction for the purposes of data collection. Various types of interview can be classified according to the degree of flexibility (Kumar, 2005). The most frequently employed interview styles are structured, semi-structured and unstructured interviews. The type of interview employed depends on the philosophy underpinning the research design. If the researcher's concern is to represent the voice of the participant only, and if they wish to limit the potential bias of their interaction with the participant as much as possible, then unstructured interviews are most appropriate. If the researcher is not unduly concerned about the impact of their presence in the data-collection process then structured or semi-structured interviews are used.

STRUCTURED INTERVIEWS

In a structured-interview format the researcher has a predetermined interview schedule. Within this interview schedule the wording and order of questions is specifically laid out. In each interview the interviewer strictly adheres to the wording and order of the interview schedule so that each interviewee is asked the same questions in the same order and style. The strength of this approach is that it allows for comparison and triangulation of data, as the interviewing process has been the same for every interviewer and interviewee. There can be more than one interviewer doing the interviewing especially if the sample population is large. Structured interviewing facilitates larger populations and the researchers may be confident that the same approach and questions have been used in each interview. A particular disadvantage with this format is that it does not allow the interviewer to deviate from the interview schedule, or to probe responses further even when the interviewee gives some insights that may develop the depth of data. This form of interviewing requires less skill than semi-structured or unstructured interviewing (Kumar, 2005).

SEMI-STRUCTURED INTERVIEWS

In semi-structured interviews the interviewer has an interview schedule in which some themes or questions are decided upon. However, during the process of the interview the interviewer may deviate from the schedule if the interviewee opens up an avenue of conversation not already catered for in the schedule. The interviewer may also probe any responses in depth as they arise. A good interviewer balances probes and deviations with their schedule as they are aware of the need to probe responses in depth but also of the importance of their schedule in ensuring the relevance of the interview. The success of semi-structured and unstructured interviews rests on the capacity of the interviewer to establish rapport and to create a safe and ethical climate within which the interview takes place.

The strength of semi-structured interviews is that they facilitate the elicitation of depth with regard to data collection. As the conversation develops between the interviewer and interviewee it may also facilitate consciousness-raising with regard to the phenomenon under investigation. For example, in health research if an interviewer asks questions with regard to lifestyle and exercise it may prompt the interviewee to critique their lifestyle behaviours. It may even encourage them to engage in a behaviour change as a result of the conversation even though their own behavioural change may not have been discussed during the interview. During the interview process the interviewer must conduct themselves in an ethical and invitational manner so that participants' experiences of research are positive and encouraging. This is not to say that if an interviewer meets with hostility (which may on a very rare occasion happen) that they may not challenge it, but they do so in a manner that does not disempower the participant or themselves.

UNSTRUCTURED INTERVIEWS

What is most attractive about unstructured interviews is that they offer the interviewer and the interviewee almost complete freedom to discuss whatever issue may arise under the theme of the investigation. However, unstructured interviews require some skill on the part of the interviewer to establish rapport and an ethical climate and also it requires skill to avoid controlling the interview with the interviewer's agenda. In unstructured interviews the interviewer is guided by the direction the interviewee takes and may use probes and ask spur-of-the-moment questions related to the discussion, but does not operate from an interview schedule. The unstructured interview actively seeks to understand the phenomenon from the participant's perspective and is committed to allowing the data to emerge itself, which then directs the focus of the research. This form of interviewing is particularly suited to grounded theory and phenomenological research.

EFFECTIVE INTERVIEWING

Key issues to be considered when planning to conduct interviews are listed below.

> Effective Interviewing
> Preparation
> Protocols
> Venue
> Recording
> Timing
> Building rapport
> Piloting
> Field notes
> Recruiting

The development of interviewing skills, particularly interpersonal skills, can greatly enhance the quality of data collection. Data that is obtained during interviews may often be weakened by inappropriate questioning, lack of effective probes, weak listening skills or weak interpersonal skills that can result in poor rapport and lack of trust on the part of the interviewee. Therefore researchers should develop their interpersonal skills and practice their interviewing techniques in order to ensure the success of their interview process.

Preparation

It is important that the researcher is familiar with the topic under investigation. This may mean conducting a comprehensive review of literature relevant to the phenomenon under investigation. This literature review will help the researcher as they develop their interview schedule. It should also assist them in the interview process as during the interaction they will be able to make connections between the data that is emerging and the themes in the literature that they have read. If using structured or semi-structured interviewing techniques the researcher should ensure that the interview schedule is relevant to the research objectives. The schedule should be clearly laid out so that the interviewer may flick their eye easily to the page without interrupting the flow of the interview or breaking eye contact for too long.

Protocols

It is important to have research principles and procedures clearly laid out at the beginning. It is helpful to have these clearly delineated on a page in the form of a letter to the participants so they are informed of the expectations of the researcher. This letter of protocol gives an indication of the general theme of the interview and the length of time the interview will take. It also explains the procedures with regard to recording of data and subsequent transcription and data use. This letter should also refer to the researcher's commitment to ethical adherence and should reiterate the principle of informed consent. Contact details for the researcher should also be provided in case the interviewee wishes to make subsequent contact. Some researchers also include a profile sheet that they fill in before the interview that has boxes to tick such as gender, age and basic demographics. This aids them later in creating anonymous profiles for research participants.

Venue

The interviewer should ensure that the venue is quiet so that the recording equipment will adequately catch the voices of the interviewer and interviewee on tape. If at all possible the interviewer should aim for a venue that is free from outside distractions. A neutral but convenient venue is also important. A venue that is not neutral may have adverse consequences on the data collected, as the interviewee may feel inhibited. If the researcher does not have a suitable venue at their disposal then they may have to opt for a public venue. In noisy hotels or cafés, voices can get lost in recording, however the reception area of a hotel may be quiet and yet may be public enough to ensure personal safety without compromising participants. The interviewer should ensure that the venue is well lit and ventilated and neither too warm (which can make people feel drowsy and lessen concentration) nor too cold (which distracts people). Often refreshments such as coffee, tea or water can help create a less formal atmosphere.

Recording

It is recommended that interviews should be recorded for accuracy. The interviewer should ensure that recording equipment is adequate but not obtrusive. Digital recording equipment enables the researcher to download the data directly onto a computer. The researcher will therefore have access to audio excerpts when presenting their research; however if transcripts are required then manual transcription must still be engaged in. Permission for recording is required prior to the interview. Participants need to be made aware of transcription procedures, data storage and subsequent disposal. Discussions with regard to anonymity are very important at this stage. A quick check prior to the interview should ensure availability of power sockets. Interviewers should also bring additional tapes and batteries. Researchers should be prepared for every eventuality with regard to the pitfalls of technology and human error. if it is possible to bring a back-up recorder this protects the interviewer in the case of equipment failure.

Timing

The interviewer should be punctual. It is important for the interviewer to be in the venue before time and to have everything set up to maximise the interaction and create the required atmosphere. The interviewer should have decided and informed the participant of the length of the interview and should adhere to their timings. Interviews generate a substantial amount of data. A one-hour long interview takes approximately nine to eleven hours to transcribe, so this may influence a researcher's decisions with regard to the length of interviews conducted.

Build rapport

Building rapport begins long before the meeting in the interview room. The process of building rapport begins at initial engagement with the research participants. How participants are invited to take part in the interview is important. If the style is invitational and participants are free to choose this is a good start; however, over-persuasion or coercion creates resistance. The researcher needs to evidence a willingness to facilitate the interviewee by agreeing mutually satisfactory timing and venues for the interviews. Full and transparent outlining of the research process is important for participants to feel empowered during the research process. Participants must be informed of their right to withdraw from the study without prejudice should they choose to do so. Maintaining eye contact and smiling is important; many interviewers are so caught up in their research process they forget the simple things like a smile to set people at ease. It is important after the interview to thank the interviewee properly and many researchers offer a token of appreciation if their budget allows. This often lets the interviewee know that they are appreciated and leaves them with a positive impression of research and of the researcher.

Pilot

It is important to pilot the interview schedule and process. Researchers may be tempted to cut corners here. They may be tempted to think that interviewing is a conversation and may not need rehearsal. However, quite the opposite is true. In piloting the researcher is testing the timing of the interview, the quality, clarity and relevance of the questioning, the venue, the recording, the probes and the establishment of rapport. The pilot test is the dry run that is imperative for successful interviewing. The researcher should ask the pilot participant to critique their interviewing technique, such as how well they put the participant at ease. They should ask the participant how they perceived the type and relevance of the questioning and they should always inquire as to whether the participant has any suggestions for improvement. In listening back over the pilot tape or reading the transcript the researcher should look for any distracting mannerisms such as the over-use of phrases or discomfort with silence which may result in the researcher's not giving the interviewee adequate time to think before answering and moving too quickly to the next question. A critical friend or colleague can support the researcher by examining the pilot results and providing constructive advice and comment. The researcher must ensure the anonymity of the pilot participant at all times.

Field notes

It is difficult to write and interview at the same time; however, when the interview is over it is often useful to have an additional tape for field notes. The interviewer can then debrief and record their field notes onto this separate tape. They can record their impressions of how the interview went, the atmosphere that was created, the points at which the interviewee became animated or resistant and the reasons why. They may also identify any points that came up that the researcher may wish to investigate further. It is important to do this straight away as in the excitement of data collection these valuable insights can get lost.

Recruiting

It can often be difficult to recruit people for interviews. People can be shy of research if they are not familiar with it. The researcher needs to approach all invitations with integrity and transparency so that potential participants can give fully informed consent. Initial recruitment is best begun with a phone call or a face-to-face invitation, as letters are often not responded to and are easier to ignore. The researcher needs to be prepared to persuade the potential participant without being forceful or exploitative. Often a clear outlining of what is involved and details of all ethical considerations, especially with regard to confidentiality and anonymity in the research representation, suffices here. If a potential interviewee has agreed to return contact and does not, it is important not to be put off by this. But it is imperative not to crowd the participant or put them off by being pushy. Give a couple of days' grace and then call again. If the potential participant then declines, the researcher should accept their decision gracefully. However, usually when the research process is explained and potential participants are informed about the ethical considerations and the importance of their contribution to the research process most people are willing to support the research.

Pitfalls to avoid

Bennett, Glatter and Levacic (1994:280) offer a somewhat crude (but helpful nonetheless) caricature of some stereotypes to avoid in interviewing. They offer five types of interviewer style to avoid:

- The ESN squirrel, who collects tapes as if they are nuts, and does not know what to do with them except play them on his hi-fi.
- The Ego Tripper, who knows in their heart their hunch is right, but just needs some interview fodder to prove it. They carefully select data to suit their purposes ignoring the rest.
- The Optimist, who plans 200 interviews with a randomly selected sample to be done in a short period of time and soon learns 200 synonyms for 'get lost'.
- The Amateur Therapist, who gets so carried away during the interview they try to resolve every emotional/social problem they encounter.
- The Guillotine, who is so intent on getting through their schedule they pay no attention to answers and cut their respondent off mid-sentence.

We would add two more:

- The Pseudo-intellectual, who is so full of their own self-importance that the question, articulated in convoluted academic-speak, takes two minutes to complete, during which time the interviewee has mentally completed their shopping list.
- The Red Herring, who veers off course at any signal and loses track of the relevance of their interview schedule. During such fishing expeditions the interviewee begins to wonder at the focus of the interview and may decide to go shark fishing instead of the agreed salmon outing.

Even though interviews may be time-consuming in terms of transcription and data analysis compared to other forms of data collection, they are perhaps the most effective data-collection tool if the researcher is aiming for depth of perception in their research. It is worth taking the time to perfect the interview schedule and the skills of interviewing as they can contribute to dynamic and person-centred research, which is most conducive to health promotion.

17
Focus Groups

Learning Outcomes:

On completion of this chapter the reader will be able to:

- define focus groups
- distinguish focus groups from group interviews
- debate the values and limitations of using focus groups
- understand the process of planning, structuring and facilitating a focus group.

INTRODUCTION

Focus groups are a qualitative data-collection method where the group conversation is the data collected. They have a long history in market research (Morgan, 1988) and they are becoming increasingly popular in health and health-promotion research because of their flexibility. Focus groups can be used as a stand-alone method or combined with other methods to triangulate data or check validity. Focus groups are particularly suited to the study of participants' attitudes, feelings, beliefs, perceptions and experiences.

DEFINING FOCUS GROUPS

Krueger and Casey (2000:5) define a focus group as a carefully planned discussion designed to obtain perceptions on a defined area of interest in a permissive and non-threatening environment.

Focus groups are distinguished from group interviews by the explicit use of the group interactions as research data (Morgan, 1988; Kitzinger, 1994, 1995). Typically the group members are asked to reflect on a series of questions or statements posed by the facilitator. Participants listen to the other participants' comments and add their own views, which may support or contradict the previous perspective. They present their own experiences and generally engage in a discussion on the topic under consideration. The objective of the focus-group interview is not to either disagree or reach a consensus, but rather to collect data on the topic within a social context where participants 'consider their own views in relation to others' (Robinson, 1999). Indeed, Millar (1996:195) cautions against the notion of facilitated or forced consensus seeking in the use of focus groups, arguing that 'any aim for consensus creates an implied pressure for conformity from the outset'. A focus-group session usually lasts between one and a half and two hours but they can be longer if the research design demands it. The number of focus groups held depends on the purpose of the group, the budget available, the target population and the achievement of data saturation. However, it is not advisable to hold serial focus groups as 'group processes, such as roles and positions of power begin to emerge' (Côté-Arsenault and Morrisson-Beedy, 2005).

THE ADVANTAGES OF USING FOCUS GROUPS

A number of distinct advantages of using focus groups were identified by Krueger (1994:37) as follows:

> The technique is a socially oriented research method capturing real life data in a social environment, possessing flexibility, high face validity, relatively low cost, potentially speedy results, and a capacity to increase the size of a qualitative study.

Other advantages of focus groups have also been identified:
- They provide opportunity for clarifying responses, following up questions and probing.
- Non-verbal communication can be observed which may complement or contradict the verbal response.
- They are a useful research tool for obtaining data from children.
- They facilitate data collection with participants who may have literacy difficulties.
- Participants who feel intimidated and unwilling to attend for individual interviews often agree to attend a focus group where they may perceive 'safety in numbers'.

The collaborative nature of focus groups can be empowering for many participants if involved in something they feel will make a difference.

THE LIMITATIONS OF USING FOCUS GROUPS

Some limitations of using focus groups have also been identified by Krueger (1994:37):

> Focus groups afford the researcher less control than individual interview, produce data that are difficult to analyse, require special skills of moderators, result in troublesome differences among groups, are based on groups that may be difficult to assemble, and must be in a conducive environment.

Additional limitations also include:
- External validity is compromised by recruitment / sampling restrictions as the group may not represent the wider population (Millar, 1996).
- Those who are not very articulate or confident may be discouraged from attending.
- They are not fully confidential or anonymous because material is shared with the other members of the group.

PLANNING THE STRUCTURE AND FACILITATION OF A FOCUS GROUP

The ultimate success of data collection often hinges upon careful planning and facilitation (Roberts, 1997). Therefore the researcher must carefully plan the structure and facilitation of the focus group. There are a number of issues to be considered including the selection of participants, selecting the moderator, devising the focus-group interview plan or schedule, piloting, ethical considerations, the setting, equipment, structuring the group, recording the data, analysing and reporting the data.

Figure 17.1 Focus group elements

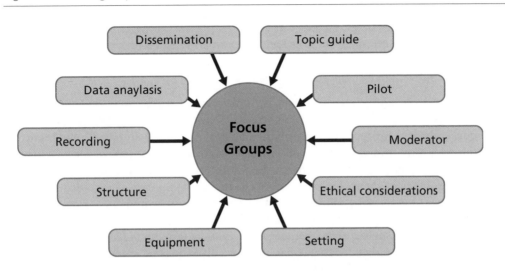

SELECTING AND RECRUITING THE TARGET-GROUP SAMPLE

Appropriateness is an essential factor when selecting a research sample in qualitative research (Morse and Field, 1996). Where the researcher carefully selects an appropriate sample, data representative of the population can be collected (Parahoo, 1997). Convenience, snowball or purposive sampling are generally used to select focus-group participants. Groups should be large enough so that diverse perspectives on a topic can be obtained and small enough so that all participants can make a significant contribution.

Generally four is considered the minimum number of participants in a focus group and twelve the upper limit. It is also generally acknowledged that there is merit in over-recruiting to focus groups. Stewart and Shamdasani (1990) suggest that at least two potential participants will not turn up. Besides issues relating to the number of participants, an equally relevant concern relates to the characteristics of the participants and issues of homogeneity. Krueger (1998) suggests recruiting seven to ten participants from similar backgrounds. Indeed most researchers recommend selecting homogenous groups (for example people from the same ethnic group, occupational group, social class, age, sex or those who share an interest in the topic under consideration, such as tobacco smoking). While this has distinct and obvious attractions, there are also situations where it can be appropriate to bring together diverse groups, for example a range of health professionals or service users, or indeed a combination of key stakeholders to achieve a broader perspective on the topic under consideration.

While combinations are potentially very useful, there are also situations where serious consideration needs to be given to the 'mix' of participants. Power differentials found in hierarchies can affect the data collected, for example nurses and patients, supervisors and employees, and should therefore be avoided. It can be difficult to recruit participants for a variety of reasons, such as time or economic considerations. To reduce the impact of factors such as these, Krueger (1998) suggests that providing meals, defraying travel costs and pointing out the opportunity to share opinions be considered as incentives as appropriate. Other possible incentives might include gift vouchers, presents or inclusion in a raffle for an attractive prize. Child minding or carer facilities may have to be provided to access some participants. The key issue here is that care must be taken to ensure that incentives are used appropriately and with due cognisance to ethical practice.

ETHICAL CONSIDERATIONS

Ethical considerations for focus groups are the same as for other methods of social research and the broad ethical principles are dealt with separately in this text. However, as a general guideline, concern should be given to participant selection, gaining access, achieving ethical approval, the conduct of the focus groups, data storage and analysis as well as dissemination. Once the format of the focus group is agreed and participants invited a letter of protocol is usually sent detailing information about the purpose of the group, the time and location. The participants should be advised that the focus group will be tape-recorded (if this is the plan) and transcribed. Written consent to participate is usually requested. Participants are usually informed of the opportunity to review the transcript to ensure that it adequately represents the content of the group discussion. Confidentiality and anonymity in relation to report writing are clarified. Participants are encouraged to keep the content of the discussion confidential and the researcher has a responsibility to protect the identity of the participants. This can be achieved by the use of pseudonyms.

TOPIC GUIDE

Once the purpose of the focus group is clear, it is usual to develop a framework by selecting topics to guide the focus group. The topics may be selected following a literature review. Bell (1993:95) asserts that:

> Where specific information is required, it is generally wise to establish some sort of structure or you may end with a huge amount of information, no time to exploit it and still without the information you need.

A topic guide differs from an interview schedule in that it serves as a reminder of the issues to be explored in the focus group. Those with little experience of moderating focus groups may prefer to develop a guide with specific questions and probes. Care is required in developing the questions and probes, which should be open-ended rather than closed and which should proceed from being broad to more focused. Open-ended questions allow the moderator to probe at a more in-depth level when appropriate, or to clear up any misunderstandings. It is important not to lead or influence the participant when probing (Parahoo, 1997). The following is an example of an open-ended question: 'How do you feel about giving smoking-cessation advice to clients?' This question encourages the person to share their feelings. Alternatively a closed question such as 'Do you like giving advice?' may encourage a yes or no response. Why-questions are best avoided as the person may feel they are being interrogated and may become defensive (Krueger, 1994). It is usual to ask no more than five major questions in an hour (Carey, 1995).

Alternatively the researcher may decide to adopt an experiential design for the focus group. This means that the researcher will design an exercise such as a brainstorming technique or a walking debate in which participants engage with the theme during the exercise rather than answering specific questions. The moderator facilitates discussion among participants as they share their responses to the exercise with the group. Thus the emphasis is on facilitation and the use of probes as issues emerge rather than on specific questions.

PILOTING FOCUS GROUPS

Baird (2000) emphasises the importance of pilot studies in supporting and enhancing the main study. However, piloting focus groups is complex due to the difficulty of separating the questions used in a focus-group interview from the environment of the focus group (Krueger, 1994). Similarly Stewart and Shamdasani (1990) advise that it is not possible to pre-test the research instrument completely as the topic guide is just one part of the procedure; the group itself and the moderator are also key elements. However, the focus group framework can be critiqued by asking experts in the field to 'review the questioning route and potential probes' (Krueger, 1994:68). The value of putting thoughts on paper and inviting others to critique is emphasised by Krueger (1994:42); who argues that 'it forces us to go beyond our individual experiences and seek the insight of colleagues'. Krueger (1994) also suggests that members of the target audience can be invited to comment on the questions or other aspects of the study and that the initial focus group can become a pilot group. Unless major changes are made this pilot discussion is included in the analysis (Krueger, 1994).

THE SETTING

By consulting with the target group, a suitable time and location can be arranged. In selecting the venue factors such as accessibility, cost implications and suitability must be considered. It is best to have a neutral venue, although focus groups can be held in people's homes, meeting rooms or other rented facilities. The room should be free from outside audio or visual distractions. Ambient factors such as the room layout, spatial arrangements, temperature and lighting are also important. Arranging the chairs with participants facing each other in a circle facilitates eye contact. A round table is also useful. The moderator must create an atmosphere that is safe, encourages interaction and appropriate disclosure and discussion. It is usual to provide refreshments such as water, tea, coffee and biscuits.

EQUIPMENT

Tape-recording of the focus group ensures accuracy of data and allows the facilitator to focus on the topic throughout the group. Video equipment can also be used, however it is important to bear in mind that this may be intimidating for the participants. The consent of the participants is required to record the session when any form of recording is used. The tape-recording equipment should be set up in advance of the interview and placed in full view of the participants, for example on the middle of a table. It is advisable to check the equipment in advance and to have a back-up in case of malfunction. Spare batteries are an essential resource to have as a standby. Other resources should be available as required, for example to record data from a brainstorming session, if appropriate. A flip-chart may be useful for summarising the discussion. Specific resources are sometimes used in focus groups, for example a card game. Such requirements should be sourced in advance.

THE ROLE OF THE MODERATOR OR FACILITATOR

The role and influence of the facilitators is seen as central to the success of the focus group (Morgan, 1993). While it is not necessary to have a professional moderator it is important to remember that the moderator requires good interpersonal and facilitation skills. This is important as the moderator's key function while the group is running is to keep the participants focused on the topic being explored. Otherwise the end product may be a fascinating and dynamic discussion that does not answer the research question. The moderator ensures that all participants have an adequate and appropriate opportunity to contribute to the discussion by skilfully controlling the dominant members and encouraging the quieter respondents to articulate their views. It is useful to have a co-facilitator to take field notes of participant dynamics. The co-facilitator can also check the recording equipment during the meeting and ensure that participants have sufficient refreshments. This person is also invaluable during the debriefing session. Where co-facilitation is used it is more likely that non-verbal cues such as body language, group dynamics and interactions will be noted and recorded, which may not be possible with a single moderator.

Structuring the focus group

The following is an example of how a focus group may be structured. The moderator usually greets the participants on arrival at the venue. Providing refreshments and engaging with the participants in casual banter for a few minutes (not related to the purpose of the session) may help them to relax. This has the added advantage of enabling the moderator to identify those individuals who are likely to be either dominant or shy in the group. The moderator may then introduce the focus group by welcoming the participants. The use of ice-breakers such as 'word bingo' can make the introduction of the participants interactive and fun.

It is important to clearly and succinctly outline the purpose of the group. Ground rules should be agreed at this stage, for example confidentiality and respect for the opinions of others. These can be written on a flip-chart and read aloud to ensure that all participants are in agreement. This creates an environment with clear boundaries and a sense of safety. The moderator must also model respect for the participants.

Once the ground rules are agreed the focus group proper begins. A range of published experiential exercises can be used in focus-group research. These are widely available in publications specific to group process and facilitation skills. If these resources are being used, follow the appropriate guidelines.

The moderator may ask the opening question, followed by supplementary questions and probes. Questions should be 'phrased simply in language that respondents understand' (Stewart and Shamdasani, 1990:65). Asking the right questions in the correct order is key to answering the research question. It is important to stress that the idea is not to ask all participants to answer the same question, rather for participants to engage in discussion.

The moderator skilfully facilitates the discussion. When the discussion is finished the moderator summarises the main points and clarifies if this perception is accurate. It is useful to invite any additional comments, suggestions, and amendments. The participants may have questions that they would like answered such as whether the researcher will furnish them with the research findings. The participants are thanked for their contribution.

A debriefing session following the focus group is an integral part of the process. In this session facilitators review and reflect on the group, suggest changes for future groups and identify initial themes.

It is advisable to make a back-up copy of the tape in case of accidental damage. The tapes should be stored appropriately and only be accessible to the research team. The tapes are transcribed verbatim. Pseudonyms can be used to protect the identity of the participants. Once transcriptions are completed the data analysis can begin.

DATA ANALYSIS

Analysis of qualitative data is indeed a complex process in which the researcher is involved in unravelling many strands and layers of meaning. Hycner (1985) suggests that researchers who transcribe tapes themselves have the opportunity to note literal statements and also non-verbal and paralinguistic communications. Analysing qualitative data is a process of bringing order to masses of collected data and it can be a 'messy, ambiguous, time consuming, creative and fascinating process' (Marshall and Rossman, 1989:112). The uncovering, articulating, elucidating and illuminating of meaning is the core purpose of data analysis (McLeod, 1999:117).

Often the data analysis becomes more coherent when the process of mapping codes begins. In mapping codes the researcher attaches a label or code to an idea or phenomenon as they come across it. As the idea or phenomenon appears again the same label or code is attached. Different labels are used for different ideas or themes. This facilitates retrieval and review of data pertaining to a particular label, code or combination of codes, at a later stage. This information can be lifted from the original version and reassembled into categories. 'This process which is called axial coding allows the researcher to fracture the data and to reassemble them in new ways' (Krueger, 1998:11). The sifting through of qualitative data has also been referred to as a process of 'funnelling' (Hope, 1994:197). 'The task is to funnel, summarise and analyse the information in order to focus on the key items' (Hope, 1994:197).

> There is an element of 'living with the data for a period until you can see the patterns within it. Having summarised them, analyse them to develop suggestions for action or ways forward on dealing with them – a process that is often better done by two or more people together.
>
> (Hope, 1994:197)

Critical friends can aid the process by reading transcripts and mapping codes which can then be compared with the codes the researcher has compiled. In the transcripts provided for the critical friend any identifying information is omitted. The critical friend must not be known to the participants to ensure as much distance and objectivity as possible. Critical friends and colleagues are important in helping the researcher explore their preferences for certain types of evidence or interpretations and can help them locate blind spots, omissions and even highlight selection bias (Davies, 1994). The analysis of focus-group data has been described as a continuum of analysis from the accumulation of raw data to the final recommendations for action (Krueger, 1998).

The Analysis Continuum

Raw Data — Description — Interpretation — Recommendation

(Krueger, 1998:27)

Raw data is basically the transcripts that present the exact statements of participants as they respond to particular topics or themes. Data reduction begins at the next stage, in which the researcher sets out a brief description of a theme followed by verbatim quotes that illustrate that theme. The descriptive style simplifies the task of the reader by providing themes and illustrative quotes. Interpretation builds on the foundations of the descriptive phase and aims to provide understanding. It is also rooted in raw data and is directly linked to the raw-data evidence from the focus group. Recommendation places greater attention on finding the multiple perspectives in the meaning of the raw data and also on various views regarding future action. Practical consequences and solution strategies are explored. Also in the recommendation phase the organisational history and traditions are explored if relevant, as they will influence decision-making (Krueger, 1998).

ANALYSIS OF GROUP PROCESSES

As group interaction is central to the use of focus groups, it is important to incorporate this as part of the data-analysis process. Stevens (1996:172) proposes a list of questions to guide the analysis of group processes:

- How closely did the group adhere to the issues presented for discussion?
- Why, how and when were related issues brought up?
- What statements seemed to evoke conflict?
- What were the contradictions in the discussion?
- What common experiences were expressed?
- Were alliances formed among group members?
- Was a particular member or viewpoint silenced?
- Was a particular view dominant?
- How did the group resolve disagreements?
- What topics produced consensus?
- Whose interests were being represented in the group?
- How were emotions handled?

When analysis is completed the findings are reported in a manner which best reflects the structure, engagement and emergent themes of the focus-group set. They are usually supported by relevant quotes.

18
Surveys

Learning Outcomes:

On completion of this chapter the reader will be able to:

- understand the uses of surveys in research
- discuss data-collection methods in survey research
- debate the principles of data analysis in survey research.

INTRODUCTION

Surveys are perhaps one of the better-known research designs. Most people are at least familiar with the term, partly due to its widespread use in the media. Reports of survey findings on a wide range of lifestyle issues and indeed sociopolitical matters are very common. Many people are 'surveyed' for their opinions or perceptions or views. A variety of types of survey as well as techniques are employed to elicit information. They are generally used for the purposes of either describing or explaining phenomena. While a number of methods of data collection are proposed in this section, including interviews, questionnaires and observational methods, the focus will be on interviews and questionnaires as the most common approaches used in surveys.

BACKGROUND AND USES OF SURVEYS

It is arguable that surveys are as old as mankind. Whether or not this is completely historically accurate, there is certainly some Biblical evidence of the use of survey methods. Weisberg *et al.* (1996) claim the earliest evidence of surveys can be found in the accounts of Moses' ascendancy to Mount Sinai and a subsequent census. In early Christian times, the story of the nativity and birth of Christ revolves around the efforts of the Romans to undertake a population census. Most established Western countries undertake a population census to aid governmental planning and indeed the Constitution of the United States requires this to happen. In the Irish context the Central Statistics Office undertakes this type of work and other governmental agencies concerned with social issues also engage in surveys as a normal part of their functioning.

Surveys have become commonplace also in the political world. George Gallup is perhaps the single name most associated with political polling. He began his work in the 1930s and his name has since become synonymous with polling of political intentions and trends. The evolution of surveys has become an integral element of social society, at least in Western countries. The use of telephone polls in news programmes is now an established element of media presentation and current affairs programmes. This is a particular form of survey aimed at gauging public opinion or responsiveness to particular questions, normally issues of media interest or controversy.

Surveys also have research uses in the study of social phenomena. They have emerged as an extremely popular research approach and are considered efficient, effective, and convenient.

While some argue that in their broadest sense, surveys are merely a means of providing information (Moser and Kalton, 1985), Fink and Kosecoff (1985:13) define a survey as 'a method of collecting information directly from people about their feelings, motivations, plans, beliefs and personal, educational and financial background'. Demonstrating the evolutionary nature of defining surveys, Arelene Fink later altered this definition to incorporate different dimensions of the approach. Fink (1995:1) included the notion of the purpose of the data-collection process. She argued that 'a survey is a system for collecting information to describe, compare, or explain knowledge, attitudes and behaviour'. This is an important distinction, in so far as surveys from a research perspective are much more than just a means of collecting descriptive information.

In their simplest form, surveys will gather information to describe phenomena, while more complex surveys are intended to describe relationships between variables including explanatory relationships. A typology described by Weisberg *et al.* (1996) is useful as a summary of the types of questions and topics that surveys are typically used to address. They include questions relating to:

- the prevalence of attitudes, beliefs and behaviours
- changes in attitudes, beliefs or behaviour over time
- group differences (between groups) in terms of their attitudes, beliefs or behaviour over time
- causal propositions about people's attitudes, beliefs or behaviour.

Clearly prevalence, individual or group changes over time or causal relationships are important in relation to attitudes, beliefs or behaviour. However, we would argue that *knowledge* and *perception* should be added to the domains of attitudes, beliefs and behaviour, as surveys are a particularly useful and common method of data collection in these fields also. Surveys are useful in capturing relationships between these domains and other variables such as personal demographics. Description or relational aspects of these domains may usefully be captured at a single point in time (cross-sectional survey) or across time (longitudinal survey).

DATA COLLECTION METHODS AND SURVEYS

Surveys are principally used to answer questions about phenomena outlined in the previous section. Surveys are closely associated with positivist traditions, and in that sense there is frequently a hypothesis to be tested in relation to any of the key domains of *attitude, belief, behaviour, knowledge or perception*. Thus surveys lend themselves to the collection of large quantities of data. Questionnaires are the most frequent means of collecting data, although they are not the only means of doing so. Figure 18.1 presents a diagrammatic representation of the main domains of survey research and the principal means of data collection as well as the central focus of issues relating to time and relationships.

Figure 18.1 Survey research: domains of interest and methods of data collection

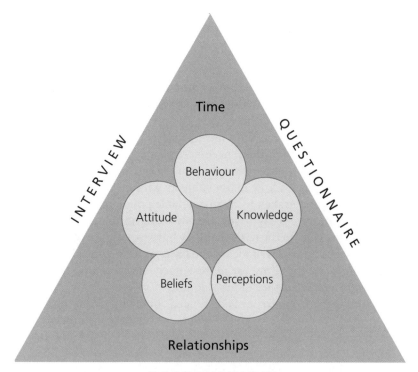

SAMPLING IN SURVEYS

A key attraction of surveys is the fact that large amounts of data can be collected efficiently and speedily. As with other forms of research, the sampling approach is dependent on the population size and the level of access the researcher has to the population. Ideally, everyone in a population should be included in surveys although for practical reasons this is frequently not possible and in terms of statistical analysis is not always necessary. An exception to this is a population census where it is necessary to include the whole population.

The sampling process is a central concern for the researcher using survey methods. When it is not possible to survey all the population of interest, it is vital that the subset chosen is representative of the overall population so that the findings from the research are generalisable.

When selecting a subset from a population, it is important to determine the sampling frame from which subjects will be drawn. A sampling frame comprises all individuals or subjects from which a sample will be selected. This may not be the complete population and the researcher needs to take account of this. For example, if undertaking a survey of the voting intentions of a population, it would seem reasonable that an electoral list may comprise the sampling frame; but an electoral list in itself may not comprise the full population, as eligible voters may have been inadvertently omitted and the eligibility status of voters may change between the time the list is compiled and the election. Therefore, in the strictest sense, findings are only generalisable to the sampling frame, thus highlighting the significance of sample selection in survey research. It is also important that the researcher using survey techniques selects their sample on the basis of the aim of the research and with due regard to relevant benefits and limitations associated with the type of sampling as this impacts on the generalisability of the findings.

SAMPLING TECHNIQUES

Sampling techniques are broadly categorised as *probability* and *non-probability* approaches. Non-probability sampling includes convenience sampling, quota sampling, purposive sampling and snowball sampling.

In convenience sampling subjects who meet predetermined criteria are included on the basis of their availability rather than necessarily being representative of the overall population. Quota sampling is a more refined form of convenience sampling. In this type of sampling, the researcher decides how many subjects who meet defined characteristics are necessary and sampling is undertaken from an available population within these parameters. Purposive sampling is more closely associated with naturalistic research. In purposive sampling, subjects are selected on the basis that they have experience of the phenomena under study. In other words a judgment is made on the basis of how 'typical' subjects are. Clearly this form of sampling does not allow for representativeness because not all members of a sampling frame stand an equal chance of inclusion.

In snowball sampling the researcher is distanced somewhat from the selection process. Members of identified groups (e.g. asylum seekers, refugees or members of the Travelling community) are approached to identify others who could be included in a study. Participants are invited on the basis of their knowledge or experience of the phenomena under investigation. Selection bias is a concern in this type of sampling, where representativeness is an important consideration.

Probability sampling is considered more desirable than non-probability sampling largely because it reduces or eliminates the possibility of selection bias. This form of sampling allows the researcher the opportunity of achieving closer representation of the overall population or sampling frame. Probability sampling adopts a systematic approach which is based on forms of randomisation. Random selection is a structured process that ensures that each individual in the sampling frame stands an equal chance of inclusion in the eventual sample. Randomisation may be *simple* or *stratified*. Although other forms of probability selection will include such approaches as *cluster sampling*, the description of approaches here is restricted to the two main forms of randomised sampling as the principles are similar.

In simple random sampling each individual stands an equal chance of inclusion. If we take an example of a survey of risky health behaviours among public servants in health-related occupations, the sampling frame might comprise all staff in the Irish Health Service Executive (HSE). Simple random sampling would mean that each employee has an equal chance of inclusion; therefore the eventual sample will be representative of all employees in this sector. This may be more than adequate if the intention is to describe such behaviours. However, if the purpose of the research is comparative or explanatory then simple random sampling may not be sufficient.

If the purpose of the study is to compare these behaviours between different occupations or grades in the HSE, then it might be more appropriate to take account of the variety of sub-populations in the employment of the HSE. In order to do so, a stratified random sample may be used. This means that samples are drawn from identified *sub-populations* using pre-determined criteria, for example occupational groups, gender or levels of organisational responsibility. These factors would be influenced by the aims and objectives of the research and would normally be informed by the existing literature in the field of enquiry. In this sampling approach the strata must be reflective of the relevant sub-groups in the sampling frame. For example among public servants there will be proportionately fewer manager grades than non-promotional grades and the stratified random sample must reflect this distribution.

DATA COLLECTION

Data collection in survey research is driven by the research question. The function of surveys is to provide information with emphasis on particular domains. Surveys are selected to either test hypotheses or to describe or explain issues of concern by answering particular questions. Questions are therefore at the heart of this form of research activity as represented in Figure 18.2.

Figure 18.2 The chain of questions in survey research

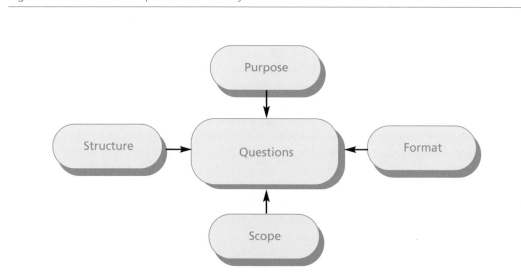

Questions will be influenced by the *format* of the study. For example, question construction and questioning technique are influenced by whether interviews, observation or questionnaires are the means of collecting the data. All questions in a survey must have a specific purpose and be directly related to the aim of the study. The means through which the information is elicited can vary in that the structure of the questions may be different. Questions may, for example, be either open or closed. This means that either the person answering the question has the scope to answer whatever they choose, in the case of open questions; or that choice is limited to a number of predetermined options in closed-question format. For example, an open question may ask 'What do you like about the current government?'. In this case, while the question is clearly seeking an answer on the performance of the current government, the person providing the information is free to answer in his or her own words. In a closed question, the choice of response is predetermined and limited to dichotomous choices of either 'yes' or 'no'; 'agree' or 'disagree'; or to multiple choices.

The format of the study also becomes an important factor in relation to the *scope* of the study. There are situations where observation rather than direct questioning is required to collect information. For example, the information required in a survey of cholesterol levels or blood-pressure readings in middle-aged males does not require the subject to answer any questions. Likewise in a survey of recording practices in medical notes, the questions would most likely be built into an audit form, observation sheet or questionnaire, to be completed by the investigator without questioning the subject concerned. Additionally, if the study involves a full national sample of 10,000 subjects, the type and format of questions will be likely to be different than in a situation where a full population comprises 200 people. The volume of data being handled as well as the complexity of analysis will be factors to be considered.

These factors should clearly influence the *structure* of the questions being asked and the questionnaire or information sheet being completed. The principles will apply irrespective of whether or not the questionnaire is being completed by an investigator or is self-administered; although clearly some issues require extra consideration when data is being collected and completed by skilled interviewers and researchers rather than by means of a self-administered questionnaire.

Both the questions and the questionnaire should be clear, easy to follow and complete. While this seems logical, it is not always the case. Only questions directly relating to the investigation should be included. Besides ethical considerations and imperatives, questions should be relevant, clear and unambiguous and the questionnaire as short as possible, so as to increase the likelihood of completion and high return rates while at the same time being sufficiently comprehensive to address the research question.

The ordering of questions or the choice of answer is influenced by the format used. It has been argued that in face-to-face or telephone interviews, where a wide variety of response options are read aloud to interviewees, they are more likely to opt for the final option. In the case of self-administered questionnaires or other written formats, respondents are more likely to opt for choices at the beginning of the list of choices (Weisberg *et al.*, 1996). Therefore the number of options becomes an issue of consideration. The wording of questions is also important. Researchers designing questionnaires or using existing ones must consider the possible meaning of questions and be aware of the danger of ambiguity in wording when posing questions as well as the possible alternatives. It is important to ensure that only one issue is being addressed by each question. Asking so-called 'double-barrelled' questions poses difficulties in terms of genuine opinions and subsequent analysis of data. An example might be 'Do you think that midwives should focus their work more on health promotion by having more antenatal classes for parents?' Clearly there is a range of complex issues within this question and it is inappropriate to attempt to address them in this manner.

A clear concern in survey research is the elimination of bias. Bias can arise when questions are structured in a manner that it is more likely to elicit one response than another. It might involve the use of emotive language. If we take an example of a complex moral issue such as euthanasia where many people hold strong beliefs, we can see where bias might be problematic in terms of getting 'true' answers. In order to address these issues, the researcher must consider whether or not to make use of existing research instruments or design new questionnaires. Making use of existing questionnaires makes sense where there is evidence to support their *validity* and *reliability*. Validity refers to whether or not the instrument measures what it says it measures and reliability refers to the capacity of the instrument to measure the same phenomenon across time. A range of levels of validity, for example content, construct and face validity, need to be addressed with new instruments, and the issue of reliability needs to be established also. This can be addressed by a pilot study and statistical testing of the instrument itself.

Completion and return of questionnaires are also matters of concern. Data will not be very useful if it is not returned for analysis. In the case of interviews, the style of accessing and agreeing interviews will have an influence on participation, completion and non-withdrawal; while in the case of self-administered questionnaires, it is extremely important that reminder letters or follow-up calls or advertising is used to enhance response rates. Response rates to postal surveys can be generally low and researchers should consider this when adopting their design. Surveys and questionnaires have become so commonplace in many societies that there can be a danger of questionnaire-fatigue or indeed forgetfulness. Both are possible explanations for non-return of questionnaires. Other considerations are the ease and cost of return. Where possible, either convenient collection points can be used or the inclusion of a stamped pre-addressed envelope should be considered. In some instances inducements are included, but this is contentious in terms of ethical considerations.

DATA ANALYSIS

Given that surveys are designed to describe or explain, there are two levels at which data can be analysed. Data analysis may be descriptive or inferential. In survey research it is normal that large quantities of data are collected, therefore the data must be in numerical format so that it can be analysed statistically. While it is possible for this to be done manually, nowadays it is normally done by computer software packages. This requires that the data is coded in such a manner that it can be inputted to the relevant statistical package and labelled appropriately. Coding involves attributing a numerical value or code to each value within each variable or element of the questionnaire. It also means ensuring that the same code or value is not attributed to multiple variables. Therefore a codebook can be very useful to ensure that every data point is coded and entered correctly. The data set should be checked and 'cleaned' against the original data so that missing values or errors in inputting are identified and rectified. It is only when this is achieved that data analysis should proceed. The level of analysis will be dependent on the research aim and objectives. Descriptive analysis may be sufficient if the aim of the survey is to describe opinions, beliefs, behaviour, knowledge and/or perceptions. Descriptive analysis allows the researcher to present data such as the mean or average score of the sample and the distribution or spread of responses. This level of analysis allows the reader to compare similarities between the sample and the overall sampling frame.

However if the aim of the research question is to discover answers to 'why' questions or causal relationships, then inferential analysis must also be undertaken. In other words, if there is a hypothesis to be tested, then descriptive analysis will be insufficient on its own. Inferential analysis allows questions of relationship to be addressed. For example, if a researcher wants to describe risky health behaviours among health professionals, then the descriptive analysis will focus on analysing the overall numbers or percentage of health practitioners who smoke or drink to excess. It will present statistical summaries of the profile of respondents; perhaps including their mean age, gender or professional background, as well as the overall size of the sample of individuals who engage in these or related activities.

This information, while important and interesting, merely describes the situation for the full sample. However, if inferential analysis is undertaken, we may be able to examine relationships between such factors as age or professional background and determine if there are differences or similarities between risky health behaviours among subsets of the sample. Thus we can draw some inferences about issues such as increased or decreased likelihood of engaging in such behaviours within or between groups in the sample. Clearly, the level of analysis, the type of analysis engaged in and the nature and strength of the inference will be dependent on a range of related factors such as the aim of the study, the nature of the data collected and the similarities of the sample to the overall population or at least the sampling frame.

19
Writing Your Research Proposal

Learning Outcomes:

On completion of this chapter the reader will be able to:

- understand the rationale for proposing research
- debate the stages of formulating a research proposal
- defend the efficacy of a research proposal.

INTRODUCTION

The research proposal can be understood as a bid or a strategy for selling one's research idea. Locke *et al.* (1993:3) identify three functions of a research proposal: communication, plan and contract. The proposal communicates the author's intentions, evidences the planning and serves as a contract between the researcher and any potential funding body. More specifically however, a research proposal is a methodical and logical plan for engaging in systematic inquiry to bring about enhanced insight with regard to the phenomenon the proposer is interested in researching. The proposal is therefore an integral aspect of any research process and it is vital for a successful research outcome.

Many research students are tempted to skimp on this aspect of their research planning, but they do so to the detriment of their research. A good research proposal not only impresses supervisors by demonstrating the author's research potential, but may also aid in any funding application. Most importantly it serves as a map for the research process and a well-planned proposal saves much time later on during the research process. A proposal serves to persuade others of the value of the research as well as demonstrating the author's knowledge of research methodologies and capability in research design. Be prepared to draft several times, for in the drafting process the refining of the research design takes place.

RESEARCH QUESTION OR AIM

A good research proposal clearly sets out a working title of the research. This is not as simple as it may sound, as crafting a research title requires much consideration. Some time must be spent refining the area of investigation, firstly by arriving at the overall research question or aim and then by focusing the research question with the aid of some objectives or research outcomes. A research objective is a 'statement of intent that specifies goals that the investigator plans to achieve in a study' (Creswell, 2005). By asking 'What exactly do I wish to find out?' and structuring the answer to this question into approximately three to five objectives the researcher can more easily identify the research focus. These objectives need to be specific to the research question, realistic and achievable.

We suggest utilising the SMART acronym when examining the objectives. They need to be Specific, Measurable, Achievable, Relevant and Timely. It is very worthwhile to spend time discussing your ideas with colleagues and a supervisor if possible as this is a significant help in the refinement of a research question. We would also suggest that draft research questions are opened to critique as other people's ideas can really support the development and refinement of research ideas into workable research questions or topics.

RATIONALE

Some consideration needs to be given to the overall rationale for undertaking the study. The value of the research needs to be established and clearly articulated in a successful research proposal. A rationale is a persuasive piece which serves to justify why the research should take place. It is often helpful to situate the research within current national or international policy. If there is a significant gap in current policy then a justification that the research is addressing this gap is helpful. However, it may also be the case that the researcher wishes to apply research procedures within a different setting, or wants to compare findings by replicating existing studies. The rationale is concerned with selling the importance of the research. The reader should be convinced of the merit of the research. This may relate, for example, to the fact that the study is timely for a specified reason, or perhaps it addresses articulated needs, answers a theoretical gap in literature, addresses a methodological issue, or the results will affect people, or will influence the improvement of practice in a profession. However, it is imperative that the author only claims what is true for the study; if the claims are grandiose, proposals are likely to be rejected.

ACCESSING LITERATURE

A research proposal should evidence that the author is cognisant of published literatures and national and international policy in their research area. It is important to keep the review of literature relevant to the research problem and situate it within the research paradigm as already described. The section on literature outlines the relevant conceptual frameworks that the author plans to engage with in support of the research process. This need not necessarily be a lengthy section but it is not a simple bulleting or listing of texts or concepts. It should be written in an integrated style and while it is theoretical in its treatment of conceptual frameworks it also serves to evidence the author's familiarity of the discourses in their chosen research area. It is also important to rely on texts within the academic field. Therefore peer-reviewed journals which represent the most recent arguments in the chosen field should be evident in the proposal as well as seminal texts in the field and key national and strategic publications, where relevant. In this section the author is integrating relevant theory and thus creating a synthesis with their research area. The literature section also provides the scope to define theoretically any relevant key concepts, thereby demonstrating the author's competency with the discourses pertaining to the research.

METHOD SECTION

We have previously distinguished between 'methodology' and methods. This section within the proposal outlines the research plan within the context of the chosen paradigm or research approach and its appropriateness for the particular area of research. In detailing the justification for the choice of paradigm, the author demonstrates their understanding of the assumptions underpinning their choice of research methodology. This section also details the methods to be employed in order to successfully address the research question. For example the author will make a clear justification of the data-collection methods proposed. These might include a questionnaire, interviews, focus groups, content analysis and so on. The important issue is that the methods proposed are justified on the basis of their relevance and may draw on theoretical justification and also citations of existing research that have used similar methods.

It is worthwhile spending some time in planning the research design. The methods proposed must fit with the research question and with the population being studied. For example if the literacy levels are unknown among the proposed population then employing a questionnaire is problematic. This section also identifies the types of sampling procedures which might be used. The researcher needs to answer the following questions:

- How many people will be selected?
- Will the researcher randomly select or stratify?
- How will the researcher access them?
- Does the researcher need permissions or help in access?
- If so how will access be negotiated?

By this stage it should be obvious that one of the imperatives of this section is that the detail of how the author plans to operationalise the research plan is the key factor to be considered. The operational issues, including instrumentation, time-line, sampling, piloting of instruments and other issues such as ethical concerns will be specific to the research being proposed. For example, a key consideration would be whether or not the researcher proposes constructing a questionnaire or alternatively utilising an existing one. If the researcher is proposing the development of a new instrument, that must be clearly justified and the processes for testing reliability and validity clearly described. It must also be evident that the researcher has the ability to design, test and use a new instrument. If the author is constructing their own instrument key questions will focus on such concerns as:

- What type of questions will it contain?
- What will influence the type of questions decided upon?
- Will demographic data be required?
- How many items or questions will be in the instrument?
- How will validity and reliability be established?
- What type of piloting procedures will be employed?

Likewise, if the use of an existing and well established instrument is being considered, it must also be evident that appropriate permissions have been sought and granted.

Clear consideration of the types and levels of data analysis should also be evident. This issue will clearly relate to the type of data collected and the volume of data to be managed. If there are small amounts of numeric data, analysis may be undertaken manually and this is also true where limited narrative data needs to be analysed. However, where large data sets are to be analysed, it is common for computer programs to be used. Clearly then, research proposals must demonstrate an appropriate level of familiarity with relevant computerised data analysis packages that might be used. For example, with questionnaires, the use of the Statistical Package for the Social Sciences (SPSS) is popular, while for qualitative data QSR, NUDIST, and NVIVO are popular packages for the sorting and analysis of data. It is extremely important that researchers spend some time exploring which type of data analysis is most appropriate and evidence it in the proposal.

It is important when dealing with methodology for the author to set the limitations of the research so that the scope is clearly evident. The population and scope of the research issue need to be clearly elucidated.

PROCEDURES AND PROTOCOLS

The procedures and protocols used should be consistent with the principles of ethical practice in research already presented. In that regard, it should be remembered that informed consent is vital in any research process. A proposal must detail how this is to be ensured. It is suggested that letters of protocol or full information sheets also be constructed for each participant detailing the requirement from the participant with regard to time, participation, recording and the general procedures that are to be adhered to by the researcher. The letter of protocol is different from the consent sheet and is for the participant to keep. It should also include contact details for the researcher so that participants may make contact should they need to clarify any issues or perhaps require support.

TIMEFRAME

A proposal should outline a realistic timeframe for the proposed research and should break this down into time for data collection, data analysis, review of relevant literature and report writing. Remember while initial collection of data (perhaps in the case of a focus group) may not be the most time-consuming element of the research process, transcription of a two-hour focus-group tape could take between sixteen and twenty hours. Inexperienced researchers are often unclear with regard to realistic timeframes and can significantly underestimate the length of time needed for the research. Therefore conversations with a supervisor or an experienced researcher are recommended as they can help with identifying the time needed.

ETHICS

In the growing culture of the importance of ethics in social research it is important to demonstrate that the author has given due consideration to the ethical issues pertaining to their proposed research. The proposal should make explicit reference to the author's plans to ensure informed consent, confidentiality, as well as issues such as the treatment of data recording and data storage. The author should address the rights of participants, as previously discussed. These will include the rights of participants to not participate or to withdraw at any point and an outline of the arrangements to cater for such situations should be included in the proposal. The author should also address other ethical requirements such as the principle of 'doing no harm'. This must be more than merely tokenistic. There should be evidence within the proposal as to what this will mean in the research practice. The inclusion of letters of protocols helps foster confidence that the researcher takes the ethical treatment of participants with the level of seriousness it deserves. Most universities, institutions and health-service providers have ethics committees which review research proposals in order to safeguard the rights of research participants. It is important to engage with these ethics committees rather then view them as a bureaucratic hurdle. Ethical approval for the research safeguards the institution as well as the researcher. When an ethics committee approves a proposal a stamp of approval is awarded to conduct the research.

DISSEMINATION

It is important that good research is disseminated. Many excellent Masters and Ph.D. research theses remain on shelves where only very few of those in the particular field may access the work. There are many ways to disseminate good research. Giving a paper at a conference is an excellent way of prompting debate and it is recommended during the research process as it may help the researcher develop their ideas. Writing an article for a professional magazine or a similar publication, which many professionals may browse through, is an excellent way of raising the discourse about one's research area among staff. Publishing an article in a peer-reviewed journal in the field should be the aim of all researchers in order to contribute to academic debate in the field. The proposal should indicate which of these options (preferably all) the author intends to use for wider dissemination of findings.

Some questions to test the efficacy of the proposal:
- Is the research question clearly identified?
- Are the research objectives SMART?
- Does the rationale justify the research well?
- Is a conceptual framework provided within which to situate the research?
- Are key authors in the field examined?
- Is the research design clearly elucidated?
- Is the sampling population and procedure outlined clearly?
- Are the research methods appropriate to the research design?
- Has data analysis been duly considered?
- Have ethical considerations been catered for?
- What ethical standards are to be applied to the research?
- Has an ethical committee perused the proposal?
- What timeframe is necessary for the research?
- Is a budget needed?
- What is the significance of the research?
- What dissemination plans are made for the research?

Once the above questions can be answered the author is in a position to commit their proposal to action with confidence. A proposal serves as a guide and is not always set in stone. As a researcher proceeds with the research they may discover the need to reshape the proposal in the light of unforeseen circumstances. It is recommended that this be done in consultation with a supervisor or critical friend in order to support the research process.

References

Addington, J., N. el-Guebaly, D. Addington and D. Hodgins (1997) 'Readiness to stop smoking in schizophrenia', *Canadian Journal of Psychiatry*, 42(1), 49–52.

Ajzen, I. and M. Fishbein (1980) *Understanding Attitudes and Predicting Behaviour*, Englewood Cliffs, NJ: Prentice Hall.

Amnesty International (2003) *Mental Illness: The Neglected Quarter*, Dublin: Amnesty International (Irish Section).

An Bord Altranais (2000) *The Code of Professional Conduct for Each Nurse and Midwife*, 2nd edn, Dublin: An Bord Altranais.

An Bord Altranais (2005) *Nursing: A Career for You*, Dublin: Nursing Careers Centre.

Anthony, P. and P. Crawford (2000) 'Service user involvement in care planning: the mental health nurse's perspective', *Journal of Psychiatric and Mental Health Nursing*, 7(5), 425–34.

Bailey, K. (2002) 'Choosing between atypical antipsychotics: weighing the risks and benefits', *Archives of Psychiatric Nursing*, 16(1), 2–11.

Baird, C. (2000) 'Taking the mystery out of research – the pilot study', *Orthopaedic Nursing*, 19(2), 42–3.

Bandura, A. (1977a) 'Self efficacy toward a unifying theory of behavioural change', *Psychological Review*, 64(2), 191–255.

Bandura, A. (1977b) *Social Learning Theory*, Englewood Cliffs, NJ: Prentice Hall.

Bandura, A. (1986) *Social Foundations of Thought and Action: A Social Cognitive Theory*, Englewood Cliffs, NJ: Prentice Hall.

Bandura, A. (1995) *Self Efficacy in Changing Societies*, New York: Cambridge University Press.

Barker, D. J. P. and G. Rose (1984) *Epidemiology in Medical Practice*, 3rd edn, Edinburgh: Churchill Livingstone.

Barrington, R. (1987) *Health, Medicine and Politics in Ireland, 1900–1970*, Dublin: Institute of Public Administration.

Barry J., B. Herity and J. Solan (1987) *The Traveller Health Status Study: Vital Statistics of Travelling People*, Dublin: The Health Research Board.

Baum, F. and C. Palmer (2002) 'Opportunity structures: urban landscape, social capital and health promotion in Australia', *Health Promotion International*, 17(4), 351–61.

Baum, F. and A. Ziersch (2003) 'Social capital', *Journal of Epidemiology and Community Health*, 57, 320–23.

Baum, F., C. Palmer, C. Modra, C. Murray and R. Bush (2000) 'Families, social capital and health' in *Social Capital and Public Policy in Australia*, ed. I. Winter, Melbourne: Australian Institute of Family Studies.

Beattie, A. (1991) 'Knowledge and control in health promotion: a test case for social policy and social theory' in *The Sociology of the Health Services*, eds. J. Gabe, M. Calnan and M. Bury, London: Routledge.

Beattie, A. (1996) 'The health promoting school: from idea to action' in *Health Promotion: Professional Perspectives*, eds. A. Scriven and J. Orme, London: Macmillan.

Beauchamp, T. and J. Childress (2001) *Principles of Biomedical Ethics*, 5th edn, Oxford: Oxford University Press.

Becker, H., ed. (1984) *The Health Belief Model and Personal Health Behaviour*, Thorofare NY: Charles B. Slack.

Beckwith, D. and C. Munn-Giddings (2003) 'Self help/mutual aid in promoting mental health at work', *Journal of Mental Health Promotion*, 2(4), 14–25.

Beeber, L. S. (1988) 'Undesirable weight gain and psychotropic medications', *Journal of Psychosocial Nursing and Mental Health Services*, 26(10), 38–40.

Bell, J. (1993) *Doing Your Research Project: A Guide for First Researchers in Education and Social Science*, 2nd edn, Buckingham, Philadelphia: Open University Press.

Benner, P. (1984) *From Novice to Expert: Excellence and power in Clinical Nursing Practice*, Menlo Park, CA: Addison-Wesley.

Benner, P. and C. Tanner (1987) 'Clinical judgement: how expert nurses use intuition', *American Journal of Nursing*, 87(1), 23–31.

Bennett, P. and R. Hodgson (1992) 'Psychology and health promotion' in *Health Promotion Disciplines and Diversity*, eds. R. Bunton and G. MacDonald, London: Routledge.

Bennett, S. and J. W. Bennett (2000) 'The process of evidence based practice in occupational therapy: informing clinical decisions', *Australian Occupational Therapy Journal*, 47, 171–80.

Bennett, N., R. Glatter and R. Levacic (1994) *Improving Educational Management through Research and Consultancy*, London: Open University Press.

Benson, A. and S. Latter (1998) 'Implementing health promoting nursing: the integration of interpersonal and health promotion', *Journal of Advanced Nursing*, 27, 100–107.

Betchel, G. A., R. Davidhizar and W. R. Spurlock (2000) 'Migrant farm workers and their families: cultural patterns and delivery in the United States', *International Journal of Nursing Practice*, 6(6), 300–306.

Bhugra, D. (2004) 'Migration and mental health', *Acta Psychiatrica Scandanavica*, 109, 243–58.

Bjornsdottir, K. (2001) 'Language, research and nursing practice', *Journal of Advanced Nursing*, 33(2), 159–66.

Black Report, *see* Department of Health and Social Security (1980).

Bloch, S. and B. Singh (1997) *Understanding Troubled Minds: A Guide to Mental Illness and Its Treatment*, Melbourne: Melbourne University Press.

Bohman, J. (2005) 'Critical theory' in *The Stanford Enclycopedia of Philosophy*, ed. E. Zalta. [Available at http://plato.stanford.edu/archives/spr2005/entries/critical-theory/]

Bouchard, C., R. J. Shepard and T. Stephens, eds. (1994) 'Physical activity, fitness and health, international proceedings and consensus statement', *Human Kinetics*, Champaign, IL: 1055.

Brennan, D. (2000) 'A Consideration of the mental health promotion policies and programs in the Eastern Health Board region, in the context of a developed theory of mental health promotion', unpublished thesis (M.Ed.), Trinity College Dublin.

Brennan Report, *see* Government of Ireland (2003b).

Brown, R. B. and S. A. Adebayo (2004) 'Perceptions of work-time and leisure-time among managers and field staff in a UK primary health care trust', *Journal of Nursing Management*, 12, 368–74.

Brown, S., H. Inskip and B. Baraclough (2000) 'Causes of the excess mortality of schizophrenia', *British Journal of Psychiatry*, 177(3), 212–17.

Buchanan, C., C. Huffman and V. Barbour (1994) 'Smoking health risk: counselling of psychiatric patients', *Journal of Psychosocial Nursing and Mental Health Services*, 32(1), 27–32.

Bury, T., and J. Mead (1998) *Evidence Based Healthcare: A Practical Guide for Therapists*, Oxford: Butterworth-Heinemann.

Callaghan, P. (2004) 'Exercise: a neglected intervention in mental health care?', *Journal of Psychiatric and Mental Health Nursing*, 11(6), 476–83.

Canadian Nurses Association (1998) 'Report on the evaluation project of the guidelines for registered nurses: working with Canadians affected by tobacco', Ottawa: Canadian Nurses Association.

Cantrell, J. (1998) 'District nurses' perceptions of health education', *Journal of Clinical Nursing*, 7(1), 89–96.

Caplan, A. (1992) 'Twenty years after. The Legacy of the Tuskegee Syphilis Study. When evil intrudes', *The Hastings Centre Report* 22(6), 29–32.

Carballo, M., J. J. Divino and D. Zerix (1998) 'Migration and health in the European Union', *Tropical Medicine and International Health*, 3(12), 936–44.

Carey, M. (1995) 'Comment: concerns in the analysis of focus group data', *Qualitative Health Research*, 5(4), 487–95.

Carey, P. (2000) 'Community health and empowerment' in *Community Health Promotion Challenges for Practice*, ed. J. Kerr, London: Balliere Tindall.

Carlisle, S. (2000) 'Health promotion and advocacy: a conceptual framework', *Health Promotion International*, 15(4), 370–78.

Carper, B. (1978) 'Fundamental ways of knowing in nursing', *Advances in Nursing Science*, 1(1), 13–23.

Carr, W. and S. Kemmis (1986) *Becoming Critical: Education, Knowledge and Action Research*, London: Falmer.

Cartwright, S. and C. L. Cooper (1997) *Managing Workplace Stress*, Thousand Oaks, CA: Sage.

Cataldo, J. K. (2001) 'The role of advanced practice psychiatric nurses in treating tobacco use and dependence', *Archives of Psychiatric Nursing*, 15(3), 107–19.

Central Statistics Office (1998) 'The demographic situation of the traveller community', *Statistical Bulletin*, December, Dublin: Stationery Office.

Central Statistics Office (2004a) *Census 2002 Report on Vital Statistics*, Dublin: Stationery Office.

Central Statistics Office (2004b) *Vital Statistics Fourth Quarter and Yearly Summary*, Dublin: Stationary Office.

Central Statistics Office (2005) *Population and Migration Estimates 2005*, Ireland: Central Statistics Office.

Centre for Health Promotion Studies (1999) *The National Health and Lifestyle Surveys (HBSC)*, Galway: Health Promotion Unit, Department of Health and Children and the Centre for Health Promotion Studies, National University of Ireland.

Centre for Health Promotion Studies (2003) *The National Health and Lifestyle Surveys (SLÁN)*, Galway: Health Promotion Unit, Department of Health and Children and the Centre for Health Promotion Studies, National University of Ireland.

Charlton, A., D. While and Y. Mochizukj (1997) 'A survey into smoking habits of nursing students', *Nursing Times*, 93(39), 58–60.

Chmiel, N. (1998) 'Psychology in the workplace' in *Psychology: A Contemporary Introduction*, eds. P. Scott and C. Spenser, Oxford: Blackwell.

Christie, A. (2003) 'Unsettling the "social" in social work: responses to asylum seeking children in Ireland', *Child and Family Social Work*, 8, 223–31.

Clark, A. M. (1998) 'The qualitative–quantitative debate: moving from positivism and confrontation to post-positivism and reconciliation', *Journal of Advanced Nursing*, 27, 1242–9.

Clark, E., T. V. Mc Cann, K. Rowe and A. Lazenbatt (2004) 'Cognitive dissonance and undergraduate nursing students' knowledge of and attitudes about smoking', *Journal of Advanced Nursing*, 46(6), 586–94.

Clarke, J. B. (1999) 'Evidence based practice: a retrograde step? The importance of pluralism in evidence generation for the practice of health care', *Journal of Clinical Nursing*, 8, 89–94.

Cloutier Laffrey, S. and G. Page (1989) 'Primary health care in public health nursing', *Journal of Advanced Nursing*, 14, 1044–50.

Cobban, S. J. (2004) 'Evidence based practice and the professionalization of dental hygiene', *International Journal of Dental Hygiene*, 2, 152–60.

Cochrane, A. L. (1979) '1931–71: a critical review with particular reference to the medical profession' in *Medicines for the Year 2000*, ed. T. Smith, London: Office of Health Economics.

Cohen, L., L. Manion and K. Morrison (2000) *Research Methods in Education*, 5th edn, London: Routledge Falmer.

Cohen, M. Z. (1987) 'A historical overview of the phenomenological movement', *IMAGE: Journal of Nursing Scholarship*, 19(1), 31–4.

Colaizzi, P. (1978) 'Psychological research as the phenomenologist views it' in *Existential Phenomenological Alternatives for Psychology*, eds. R. S. Valle and M. King, New York: Oxford University Press, 48–71.

Combat Poverty Agency (2003) *Annual Report*, Dublin: Combat Poverty Agency.

Cooper, C., S. Sloan and S. Williams (1988) *Occupational Stress Indicator: Management Guide*, Windsor: NFER–Nelson.

Cooper, J. (1997) 'The perceived value of occupational health', *Occupational Health Review*, 70, 25–8.

Cort, E., J. Attenborough and J. P. Watson (2001) 'An initial exploration of community mental health nurses' attitudes to an experience of sexuality-related issues in their work with people experiencing mental health problems', *Journal of Psychiatric and Mental Health Nursing*, 8(6), 489–99.

Côté-Arsenault, D. and D. Morrisson-Beedy (2005) 'Focus on research methods. Maintaining your focus in focus groups: avoiding common mistakes', *Research in Nursing and Health*, 28, 172–9.

Coughlan, D. and T. Brannick (2005) *Doing Research in Your Own Organisation*, 2nd edn, London: Sage.

Cox, E. (1995) *A Truly Civil Society*, Sydney: ABC Books.

Cox, S. (1985) 'Women's work: women's health', *Occupational Health: A Journal for Occupational Health Nurses* (London), 37(11), 504–13.

Cox, T. and E. Ferguson (1994) 'Measurement of the subjective work environment', *Work and Stress*, 8(2), 98–109.

Crehan, M. (2001) 'Suicide prevention: a shared endeavour', *Journal of Health Gain*, 5(4), 16–17.

Creswell, J. (2005) *Educational Research: Planning, Conducting and Evaluating Quantitative and Qualitative Research*, 2nd edn, New Jersey: Pearson Prentice Hall.

Cronbach, L. J. (1975) 'Beyond the two disciplines of scientific psychology', *American Psychologist*, 30(2), 116–27.

Curry, J. (1998) *Irish Social Services*, 3rd edn, Dublin: Institute of Public Administration.

Dahlgren, G. and M. Whitehead (1991) *Policies and Strategies to Promote Social Equality in Health*, Stockholm: Institute of Futures Studies.

Dalack, G. W. and A. H. Glassman (1992) 'A clinical approach to help psychiatric patients with smoking cessation', *Psychiatric Quarterly*, 63(1), 27–39.

Davidson, N., S. Skull, D. Burgner, P. Kelly, S. Raman, D. Silove, Z. Steel, R. Vora and M. Smith (2004) 'An issue of access: delivering equitable health care for newly arrived refugee children in Australia', *Journal of Paediatric Child Health*, 40, 569–75.

Davidson, S., F. Judd, D. Jolley, B. Hocking and S. Thompson (2001a) 'Cardiovascular risk factors for people with mental illness', *Australian and New Zealand Journal of Psychiatry*, 35(2), 196–202.

Davidson, S., F. Judd, D. Jolley, B. Hocking, S. Thompson and B. Hyland (2001b) 'Risk factors for HIV/AIDS and hepatitis C among the chronic mentally ill', *Australian and New Zealand Journal of Psychiatry*, 35(2), 203–9.

Davies, R. (1994) 'Coming to terms with research', unpublished course materials, Centre for Applied Research in Education, Norwich.

Davis, S. M. (1995) 'An investigation into nurses' understanding of health education and health promotion within a neuro-rehabilitation setting', *Journal of Advanced Nursing*, 21, 951–9.

Deasy, C. (2005) 'Health promotion in mental health nursing: an exploratory study of the perceptions of mental health nurses in one geographical region', unpublished thesis (M.A. Health Education Promotion), University of Limerick.

Department of Health (1984) *The Psychiatric Services: Planning for the Future*, Dublin: Stationery Office.

Department of Health (1986) *Health: The Wider Dimensions*, Dublin: Stationery Office.

Department of Health (UK) (2001) *Making It Happen: A Guide to Delivering Mental Health Promotion*, London: Department of Health.

Department of Health and Human Services (US) (1980a) *Healthy People: The Surgeon General's Report on Health Promotion and Disease Prevention*, Rockville, MD: Department of Health and Human Services.

Department of Health and Human Services (US) (1980b) *Promoting Health/Preventing Disease: Objectives for the Nation*, Rockville, MD: Department of Health and Human Services.

Department of Health and Human Services (US) (1990) *Healthy People 2000: National Health Promotion and Disease Prevention Objectives*, Rockville, MD: Department of Health and Human Services.

Department of Health and Human Services (US) (2000) *Healthy People 2010: Understanding and Improving Health*, Rockville, MD: Department of Health and Human Services.

Department of Health and Social Security (UK) (1980) *Inequalities in Health: Report of a Research Working Group Chaired by Sir Douglas Black* [Black Report], London: DHSS.

Department of Human Services (1995) *Victoria's Health: Second Report on the Health Status of Victorians*: Victoria: Public Health Division, Department of Human Services.

Department of the Taoiseach (2004) *Sustaining Progress 2003–2005: Progress Report on Special Initiatives*, Dublin: Department of the Taoiseach.

Dickens, G. L., J. H. Stubbs and C. M. Haw (2004) 'Smoking and mental health nurses: a survey of clinical staff in a psychiatric hospital', *Journal of Psychiatric and Mental Health Nursing*, 11(4), 445–51.

DoHC (1993) *The Years Ahead: A Policy for Older People*, Dublin: DoHC.

DoHC (1994) *Shaping a Healthier Future: A Strategy for Effective Healthcare in the 1990s*, Dublin: Stationery Office.

DoHC (1995) *A Health Promotion Strategy: Making the Healthier Choice the Easier Choice*, Dublin: DoHC.

DoHC (1998a) *Report of the Commission on Nursing: A Blueprint for the Future*, Dublin: Stationery Office.

DoHC (1998b) *Report of the National Task Force on Suicide*, Dublin: Stationery Office.

DoHC (1999) *Building Healthier Hearts: The Report of the Cardiovascular Health Strategy Group*, Dublin: DoHC.

DoHC (2000) *The National Health Promotion Strategy 2000–2005*, Dublin: Stationery Office.

DoHC (2001a) *Adolescent Health Strategy*, Dublin: Stationery Office.

DoHC (2001b) *Quality and Fairness: A Health System for You*, Dublin: Stationery Office.

DoHC (2001c) *Report of the Inspector of Mental Hospitals for the Year Ending 31st December 2000*, Dublin: Stationery Office.

DoHC (2001d) *The Health of Our Children*, Dublin: Stationery Office.

DoHC (2002) *Traveller Health: A National Strategy 2002–2005*, Dublin: Stationery Office.

DoHC (2003a) *Annual Report*, Dublin: Stationery Office.

DoHC (2003b) *Nurses' and Midwives' Understanding and Experiences of Empowerment in Ireland, Final Report*, Dublin: Stationery Office.

DoHC (2003c) *Report of the Inspector of Mental Hospitals for the Year Ending December 2003*, Dublin: Stationery Office.

DoHC (2003d) *Report of the National Task Force on Medical Staffing*, Dublin: DoHC.

DoHC (2004a) *Better Health through Prevention; 4th Annual Report of the Chief Medical Officer*, Dublin: DoHC.

DoHC (2004b) *European Home and Leisure Accident Surveillance System; Report for 2002*, Dublin: Stationery Office.

DoHC (2004c) *Review of the National Health Promotion Strategy*, Dublin: Stationery Office.

Downie, R. S., C. Tannahill and A. Tannahill (1996) *Health Promotion Models and Values*, 2nd edn, Oxford: Oxford University Press.

Duasco, M. J. and P. Cheung (2002) 'Issues and innovations in nursing practice: health promotion and lifestyle advice in general practice: what do patients think?', *Journal of Advanced Nursing*, 39(5), 472–83.

Dubrin, A. J. (1978) *Human relations: A Job-orientated Approach*, New York: Reston Publishing Co.

Duxbury, L. and C. Higgins (2001) 'Work-life balance in the new millennium: where are we? where do we need to go?' Canadian Policy Research Network discussion paper no. 3, Ottawa: CPRN.

Earle, S. (2001) 'Disability, facilitated sex and the role of the nurse', *Journal of Advanced Nursing*, 36(3), 433–40.

Eckstein, S. (1998) *Manual for Research Ethics Committees*, Cambridge: Cambridge University Press / Royal College of Nursing.

Edward, D. and P. Burnard (2003) 'A systematic review of stress and stress management interventions for mental health nurses', *Journal of Advanced Nursing*, 42(2), 169–200.

Elliott, J. (1991) *Action Research for Educational Change*, Buckingham: Open University Press.

Elmore, R. (1989) 'Backward mapping' in *Policies for the Curriculum*, eds. B. Moon, P. Murphy and J. Raynor, London: Open University Press.

Falk-Rafael, A. (1999) 'The politics of health promotion: influences on public health promoting nursing practice in Ontario, Canada from Nightingale to the nineties', *Advances in Nursing Science*, 22(1), 23–41.

Falk-Rafael, A. (2001) 'Empowerment as a process of evolving consciousness: a model of empowered caring', *Journal of Advanced Nursing Science*, 24(1), 1–16.

Festinger, L. (1957) *A Theory of Cognitive Dissonance*, Stanford, CA: University Press.

Fleming, S., C. Kelleher and M. O Connor (1997) 'Eating patterns and factors influencing likely change in the workplace in Ireland', *Health Promotion International*, 12, 187–96.

Finfgeld, D. L., S. Wongvatunyu, V. S. Conn, V. Grando and C. L. Russell, (2003) 'Health belief model and reversal theory: a comparative analysis', *Journal of Advanced Nursing*, 43(3), 288–97.

Fink, A. (1995) *The Survey Handbook*, Thousand Oaks: Sage.

Fink, A. and J. Kosecoff, (1985) *How To Conduct Surveys: A Step by Step Guide*, Beverly Hills: Sage.

Fontaine, K. L. (2003) *Mental Health Nursing*, 5th edn, New Jersey: Prentice Hall.

Foucault, M. (1997) *Ethics, Subjectivity and Truth*, ed. P. Rabinow, London: Penguin.

Fox, K. R. (2000) 'Physical activity and mental health promotion: the natural partnership', *International Journal of Mental Health Promotion*, 2(1), 4–12.

Freire, P. (1970) *Pedagogy of the Oppressed*, New York: The Continuum Publishing Press.

French, P. (1999) 'The development of evidence based nursing', *Journal of Advanced Nursing*, 29(1), 72–8.

Friedli, L. and C. Dardis (2002) 'Not all in the mind: mental health service user perspectives on physical health', *Journal of Mental Health Promotion*, 1(1), 36–46.

Fuimano, J. (2005) 'Before nurse leaders can create a work/life balance, they must first define their ideal scenario', *Nursing Management*, 36(5), 23–5.

Furber, C. M. (2000) 'An exploration of midwives' attitude to health promotion', *Midwifery*, 16(4), 314–22.

Galinsky, E. (1999) *Ask the Children: What America's Children Really Think about Working Parents*, New York: William Morrow and Company, Inc.

Gall, M., W. Borg and J. Gall (1999) *Educational Research: An Introduction*, 6th edn, New York: Longman.

Geary, T. and P. Mannix McNamara (2005) *The Involvement of Male Post-primary Teachers in Relationships and Sexuality Education: An Exploratory Study of Attitudes and Perceptions*, Limerick: University of Limerick.

Gerrish, K. and J. Clayton (2004) 'Promoting evidence based practice: an organisational approach', *Journal of Nursing Management*, 12, 114–23.

Gillon, R. (1986) *Philosophical Medical Ethics*, Chichester: Wiley.

Gilman, S. E., I. Kawachi, G. M. Fitzmaurice and S. L. Buka (2002) 'Socioeconomic status in childhood and the lifetime risk of major depression', *International Journal of Epidemiology*, 31(2), 359–67.

Glaser, B. (2005) *Grounded Theory Perspective III: Theoretical Coding*, Mill Valley, CA: Sociology Press.

Glaser, B. and A. Strauss (1967) *The Discovery of Grounded Theory: Strategies for Qualitative Research*, New York: Aldine Publishing.

Goodman, R., A. Steckler and M. Kegler (2002) 'Mobilising organisations for health enhancement: theories of organisational change' in *Health Behaviour and Health Education: Theory, Research and Practice*, 2nd edn, ed. K. Glanz, San Francisco: Jossey-Bass.

Gopalaswamy, A. K. and R. Morgan (1985) 'Too many chronic mentally disabled patients are too fat', *Acta Psychiatrica Scandinavica*, 72(3), 2548.

Government of Ireland (1966) *Report of the Commission of Inquiry on Mental Illness*, Dublin: Stationery Office.

Government of Ireland (1970) *Report on the Industrial and Reformatory Schools System*, Dublin: Stationery Office.

Government of Ireland (1974) *Commission of Inquiry on Mental Handicap*, Dublin: Stationery Office.

Government of Ireland (1988) *The Years Ahead: A Policy for the Elderly: Report of the Working Party on Services for the Elderly*, Dublin: Stationery Office.

Government of Ireland (1990) *Needs and Abilities: A Policy for the Intellectually Disabled / Report of the Review Group on Mental Handicap Services*, Dublin: Stationery Office.

Government of Ireland (1995) White Paper: *Charting Our Education Future*, Dublin: Stationery Office.

Government of Ireland (2000) *Equal Status Act*, Dublin: Stationery Office.

Government of Ireland (2003a) *Audit of Structures and Functions in the Health System* [The Prospectus Report], Watson Wyatt Worldwide on behalf of the Department of Health and Children, Dublin: Stationery Office.

Government of Ireland (2003b) *Commission on Financial Management and Control Systems in the Health Service* [The Brennan Report], Dublin: Stationery Office.

Government of Ireland (2003c) *National Action Plan against Poverty and Social Exclusion*, Dublin: Stationery Office.

Government of Ireland (2003d) *Sustaining Progress: Social Partnership Agreement 2003–2005*, Dublin: Stationery Office.

Graham, H. and G. Derl, (1999) 'Patterns and predictors of smoking cessation among British women', *Health Promotion International*, 14(3), 231–40.

Graw, B. (1979) 'Process questions: an aid to completing the learning cycle' in *The Annual Handbook for Group Facilitators*, eds. J. Pfeiffer and J. Jones, California: University Associates Publishers.

Gray, P. (2000) *Mental Health in the Workplace: Tackling the Effects of Stress*, London: Mental Health Foundation.

Gray, R., E. Brewin, J. Noak, J. Wyke-Joseph and B. Sonik (2002) 'A review of the literature on HIV infection and schizophrenia: implications for research, policy and clinical practice', *Journal of Psychiatric and Mental Health Nursing*, 9(4), 405–9.

Green, L. W. and J. M. Raeburn (1988) 'Health promotion, what is it? What will it become?', *Health Promotion*, 3(2), 151–9.

Grinyer, A. (2001) 'Ethical Dilemmas in non-clinical health research', *Nursing Ethics*, 8(2), 123–32.

Grix, J. (2004) *The Foundations of Research*, Basingstoke: Palgrave Macmillan.

Guba, E. G. (1990) *The Paradigm Dialog*, London: Sage.

Gunnarsdottir, S. and K. Bjornsdottir (2003) 'Health promotion in the workplace: the perspective of unskilled workers in the hospital setting', *Scandinavian Journal of Caring Science*, 17, 66–73.

Haase, J. E. and S. Taylor Myers (1998) 'Reconciling paradigm assumptions of qualitative and quantitative research', *Western Journal of Nursing Research*, 10(2), 128–37.

Habermas, J. (1972) *Knowledge and Human Interests*, tr. J. Shapiro, London: Heinemann.

Handy, C. (1976) *Understanding Organisations*, London: Penguin.

Harris, E. C. and B. Baraclough (1998) 'Excess mortality of mental disorder', *British Journal of Psychiatry*, 173, 11–53.

Harris, E. E. (1966) *Ethical Issues in Health Care*, St Louis: C. V. Mosby.

Harrison (2004) 'Health promotion and politics' in *Health Promotion: Disciplines, Diversity and Developments*, 2nd edn, eds. R. Bunton and G. Macdonald, London: Routledge.

Health Education Authority (1997) *Mental Health Promotion: A Quality Framework*, London: Health Education Authority.

Heidegger, M. (1962) *Being and Time*, trs. J. Macquarrie and E. Robinson, San Fransisco: Harper and Row.

Henderson, V. (1991) *The Nature of Nursing: A Definition and Its Implications for Practice, Research and Education*, New York: Macmillan.

Herrman, H. (2001) 'The need for mental health promotion', *Australian and New Zealand Journal of Psychiatry*, 35(6), 709–15.

Hewinson, A. (1995) 'Nurses' power in interactions with patients', *Journal of Advanced Nursing*, 21(1), 75–82.

Hewitt, J. (2002) 'A critical review of the arguments debating the role of the nurse advocate', *Journal of Advanced Nursing*, 37(5), 439–45.

Hjelm, K. G., K. Bard, P. Nyberg and J. Apelqvist (2005) 'Beliefs about health and diabetes in men of different ethnic origin', *Journal of Advanced Nursing*, 50(1), 47–59.

HM Treasury and Department of Trade and Industry (2003) *Balancing Work and Family Life: Enhancing Choice and Support for Parents*, London: HM Treasury Stationery Office.

Hochbaum, G. (1958) *Public Participation in Medical Screening Programmes: A Socio-psychological study*, Public Health Services Publication no. 572, Washington DC: US Government Printing Office.

Hodge, M. (2000) 'It's not just working parents who want work-life balance', Department of Trade and Industry Press Release, September 7. [Available at http://www.dti.gov.uk/work-lifebalance/press_005_c.html]

Hodgson, R. J. (1996) Editorial: 'Mental health promotion', *Journal of Mental Health*, 5(2).

Hope, A. and C. Kelleher (1995) *Health at Work*, Galway: Centre for Health Promotion Studies, University College Galway.

Hope, A., C. Dring and J. Dring (2004) *College Lifestyle and Attitudinal National Survey*, Galway: National University of Ireland.

Hope, A., N. Kelleher and M. O Connor (1998) 'Lifestyle practices and the health promoting environment of hospital nurses', *Journal of Advanced Nursing*, 28(2), 438–47.

Hope, P. (1994) 'Diagnosis: data collection and feedback in consultancy' in N. Bennett, R. Glatter and R. Levacic, *Improving Educational Management through Research and Consultancy*, London: Paul Chapman Publishing.

Horkheimer, M. (1982) *Critical Theory*, New York: Seabury Press.

Houlihan, G. (1999) 'The evaluation of the stages of change model for use in the counselling of clients undergoing predictive testing for Huntington's disease', *Journal of Advanced Nursing*, 29(5), 1137–43.

Hughes, J. and W. Sharrock (1997) 'Positivism and the language of the social researcher' in *Philosophy of Social Research*, 3rd edn, J. Hughes and W. Sharrock, Longman, 42–75 and 210–16.

Hussey, D. (1995) *How to Manage Change*, London: Kogan Page.

Hycner, R. (1985) 'Some guidelines for the phenomenological analysis of interview data', *Human Studies*, 8, 279–303.

Hyland, B., F. Judd, S. Davidson, D. Jolley and B. Hocking (2003) 'Case manag
to the physical health of their patients', *Australian and New Zealan*
Psychiatry, 37(6), 710–14.

Iribarren, C., R. V. Luepker, P. G. McGovern, D. K. Arnett and H. Blackburn (1. . . ,
year trends in cardiovascular disease risk factors in the Minnesota Heart Survey. Are
socioeconomic differences widening?', *Archives of Internal Medicine*, 157(8), 873–81.

Irish Heart Foundation (2005) *Happy Heart at Work News*, 1(2).

Irish Sudden Infant Death Association (1999) *National Sudden Infant Death Register*
Report, Dublin: Irish Sudden Infant Death Association.

Irish Universities Nutrition Alliance (2001) *The North South Ireland Food Consumption*
Survey. [Available at http://www.iuna.net/survey_contents.htm]

Irwin, R. (1997) 'Sexual health promotion and nursing', *Journal of Advanced Nursing*, 25(1),
170–77.

Jackson, S., V. Varon and S. Cleverly (1986) *Public Health Practitioner Perspectives on*
Empowerment: Definition, Strategies and Indicators, New York: Community Health
Promotion Research Unit.

Jackson-Triche, M. E., J. Greer Sullivan, K. B. Wells, W. Rogers, P. Camp and R. Mazel
(2000) 'Depression and health-related quality of life in ethnic minorities seeking care in
general medical settings', *Journal of Affective Disorders*, 58(2), 89–97.

Janz, N. and M. Becker (1984) 'The health belief model: a decade later', *Health Education*
Quarterly, 11, 1–47.

Jasper, M. A. (1994) 'Issues in phenomenology for researchers of nursing', *Journal of*
Advanced Nursing, 19(2), 309–14.

Johnson, J., L. Green, C. I. Frankish, D. MacLean and S. Stachenko (1996) 'A dissemination
research agenda to strengthen health promotion and disease prevention', *Canadian*
Journal of Public Health, 87(2), 5–11.

Johnson, M. E. (2000) 'Heidegger and meaning: implications for phenomenological
research', *Nursing Philosophy*, 1(2), 134–46.

Jones, A. (2003) *About Time For Change*, London: The Work Foundation in association with
Employers for Work-Life Balance.

Jones, L. J. (1994) *The Social Context of Health and Health Work*, Basingstoke: Palgrave.

Karch, B. (2000) 'A case for physical activity in health promotion', *Health Promotion:*
Global Perspectives, 2(6), 1.

Kelleher, C. (1998) 'Evaluating health promotion in four key settings' in *Quality, Evidence*
and Effectiveness in Health Promotion, eds. J. K. Davies and G. MacDonald, London:
Routledge.

Kelly, A., M. Carvalho and C. Teljeur (2003) *A 3-Source Capture Recapture Study of the*
Prevalence of Opiate Use in Ireland 2000 to 2001, Dublin: Department of Community
Health and General Practice, Trinity College Dublin. [Available at www.nacd.ie]

Kemmis, S. and R. McTaggart (1982) *The Action Research Planner*, Geelong: Deakin
University Press.

Kendall, R. E. (1983) 'Alcohol and suicide', *Substance and Alcohol Actions/Misuse*, 4(2–3),
121–7.

Kennedy, B. P., I. Kawachi and D. Prothrow-Stith (1996) 'Income distribution and mortality:
cross sectional ecological study of the Robin Hood index in the United States', *British*
Medical Journal, 312(7037), 1004–7.

King, L., P. Hawe and M. Wise (1998) 'Making dissemination a two way process', *Health*
Promotion International, 13(3), 237–44.

Kitzinger, J. (1994) 'The methodology of focus groups: the importance of interaction between research participants', *Sociology of Health and Illness*, 16(1), 103–21.

Kitzinger, J. (1995) 'Introducing focus groups', *British Medical Journal*, 311(7000), 299–302.

Kitzinger J. and R. S. Barbour (1999) 'Introduction to the challenge and promise of focus groups' in *Developing Focus Group Research: Politics, Theory and Practice*, eds. R. S. Barbour and J. Kitzinger, London: Sage, 1–20.

Kolb, D. (1984) *Experiential Learning: Experience as the Source of Learning and Development*, London: Prentice Hall.

Krueger, R. A. (1994) *Focus groups: A Practical Guide for Applied Research*, London: Sage.

Krueger, R. (1998) 'Analysing and reporting focus group data' in D. Morgan and R. Krueger, *The Focus Group Kit*, London: Sage.

Krueger, R. A. (1998) *Focus groups: A Practical Guide for Applied Research*, 2nd edn, California: Sage.

Krueger, R. A. and M. A. Casey (2000) *Focus Groups: A Practical Guide for Applied Research*, Thousand Oaks, CA: Sage.

Kuhn, T. (1977) *The Essential Tension: Selected Studies in Scientific Tradition and Change*, Chicago: University of Chicago Press.

Kuhn, T. S. (1970) *The Structure of Scientific Revolutions*, 2nd edn, Chicago: University of Chicago Press.

Kumar, P. and R. Ghadially (1989) 'Organizational Politics and its effects on members of organizations', *Human Relations*, 42(4), 305–14.

Kumar, R. (2005) *Research Methodology: A Step-By-Step Guide for Beginners*, 2nd edn, London: Sage.

Kunitz, S. (2000) 'Accounts of social capital: the mixed health effects of personal communities and voluntary groups' in *Poverty, Inequality and Health: An International Perspective*, eds. D. Leon and G. Walts, Oxford: Oxford University Press.

Kvale, S. (1996) *Interviews*, London: Sage.

La Ferla, A. (1993) Foreword in *Psychosocial and Organizational Hazards*, eds. T. Cox and S. Cox, 5th edn, Copanhagen: World Health Organization (Europe).

LaLonde, M. (1974) *A New Perspective on the Health of Canadians: A Working Document*, Canada: Department of Health and Welfare.

Lasser, K., J. Wesley-Boyd, S. Woolhandler, D. U. Himmelstein, D. Mc Cormick and D. H. Bor (2000) 'Smoking and mental illness: a population based prevalence study', *Journal of the American Medical Association*, 284(20), 2606–10.

Lawn, S. J., R. G. Pols and J. G. Barber (2002) 'Smoking and quitting: a qualitative study with community living psychiatric clients', *Social Science and Medicine*, 54(1), 93–104.

Leedy, P. and J. Ormond (2005) *Practical Research, Planning and Design*, 8th edn, New Jersey: Pearson, Prentice Hall.

Le Touze, S. (1996) 'Health promotion in general practice: the views of staff', *Nursing Times*, 92, 32–3.

Lewin, K. (1946) Action research and minority problems', *Journal of Social Issues*, 2, 34–46.

Lewin, K. (1951) *Field Theory and Social Science: Selected Theoretical Papers*, London: Tavistock Publications, Routledge and Kegan Paul.

Lewin, K. (1958) 'Group decisions and social change' in *Readings in Social Psychology*, eds. G. Swanson, T. Newcomb and E. Hartley, New York: Holt Rineheart & Winston.

Lewis, J. and E. Scott (1997) 'The sexual education needs of those disabled by mental illness', *Psychiatric Rehabilitation Journal*, 21, 164–7.

Lewis, S. and R. Bor (1994) 'Nurses' knowledge of and attitudes towards sexuality and the relationship of these with nursing practice', *Journal of Advanced Nursing*, 20(2), 251–9.

Littlewood, J. and I. Parker (1992) 'Community nurses' attitude to health promotion in one regional health authority', *Health Education Journal*, 51(2), 87–9.

LoBionda-Wood, G. and J. Harber (1998) *Nursing Research Methods Critical Appraisal and Utilization*, Missouri: Mosby.

Locke, L., W. Spirduso and S. Silverman (1993) *Proposals that Work*, 3rd edn, Newbury Park, CA: Sage.

Luft, S. (2005) 'Husserl's concept of the "transcendental person"; another look at the Husserl-Heidegger relationship', *International Journal of Philosophical Studies*, 13(2), 141–77.

Lukes, S. (1974) *Power: A Radical View*, London: Macmillan.

Lynch, J., G. A. Kaplan, R. Salonen and J. T. Salonen (1997) 'Socioeconomic status and progression of carotid atherosclerosis. Prospective evidence from the Kuopio Ischemic Heart Disease Risk Factor Study', *Arteriosclerosis, Thrombosis and Vascular Biology*, 17(3), 513–9.

Maben, J. and J. Macleod Clark (1995) 'Health promotion: a concept analysis', *Journal of Advanced Nursing*, 22(6), 1158–65.

Macdonald, E. B., K. A. Ritchie, K. J. Murray and W. H. Gilmour (2000) 'Requirements for occupational medicine based training in Europe: a Delphi study', *Occupational Environmental Medicine*, 57, 98–105.

MacDonald, M. A. (2004) 'From miasma to fractals: the epidemiology revolution and public health nursing', *Public Health Nursing*, 21(4), 380–91.

Macleod Clark, J., S. Haverty and S. Kendall (1990) 'Helping people to stop smoking: a study of the nurse's role', *Journal of Advanced Nursing*, 15(3), 357–63.

Mannix McNamara, P. (2004) 'Workplace bullying: critical reflections and the problematics of culture', keynote address, International Workplace Bullying Conference, Adelaide, April 2004.

Mannix McNamara, P. (2005a) 'Educational workplaces: culture, power and pedagogy – a critical perspective', keynote address, Australian Educational Union, Occupational Health and Safety at Work Conference, Adelaide, August 2005.

Mannix McNamara, P. (2005b) 'How do I improve my practice as a professional educator by developing my critical awareness of how I pedagogise knowledge within the academy?', paper delivered at National Educational Studies Association of Ireland Conference, Cork, March 2005.

Marshall. C. and G. Rossman (1989) *Designing Qualitative Research*, London: Sage.

Mason, R. (1993) *Empowerment and Annotated Bibliography*, Report Series no. 93–03, North York, Ontario: Community Health Promotion Research Unit.

Maville, J. A. and C. G. Huerta (2002) *Health Promotion in Nursing*, USA: Delmar.

McAuliffe, E. and L. Joyce (1998) *A Healthier Future? Managing Healthcare in Ireland*, Dublin: Institute of Public Administration.

McCubbin, M. (2001) 'Pathways to health, illness and well-being: from the perspective of power and control', *Journal of Community and Applied Social Psychology*, 11, 75–81.

McEvoy, R. and N. Richardson (2004) *Men's Health in Ireland: A Report from the Men's Health Forum in Ireland*, Belfast: Men's Health Forum Ireland Publishing.

Mc Haffie, H. (1994) 'HIV and AIDS: a survey of nurse education in the United Kingdom', *Journal of Advanced Nursing*, 20(3), 552–9.

McKenna, H. P., S. Ashton and S. Keeney (2002) 'Barriers to evidence based practice in primary care', *Journal of Advanced Nursing*, 45(2), 178–89.

McKevitt, D. (1998) 'Irish healthcare policy: legislative strategy or administrative control?' in *A Healthier Future? Managing Healthcare in Ireland*, eds. E. McAuliffe and L. Joyce, Dublin: Institute of Public Administration.

McKenzie, J. F. and J. L. Smeltzer (2001) *Planning, Implementing and Evaluating Health Promotion Programmes: A Primer*, 2nd edn, Boston: Allyn and Bacon.

McKinsey & Company, Inc. (1970–71) *Towards better Healthcare Management in the Health Board*, Dublin: McKinsey & Company, Inc.

McLeod, J. (1999) *Practitioner Research in Counselling*, London: Sage.

Mc Mahon, A., C. Kelleher, E. Duffy and G. Helly (2001) *An Evaluation of the Happy Heart at Work Programme*, Centre for Health Promotion Studies NUI Galway on behalf of the Irish Heart Foundation.

McNamara, C. (2005) [Available at http://www.managementhelp.org/org_thry/org_defn.htm]

McNiff, J. (2002) *Action Research: Principles and Practice*, London: Routledge Falmer.

McNiff, J., P. Lomax and J. Whitehead (2003) *You and Your Action Research Project*, 2nd edn, London: Routledge Falmer.

Meadows, G., K. Stasser, K. Moeller-Saxone, B. Hocking, J. Stanton and P. Kee (2001) 'Smoking and schizophrenia: the development of collaborative management guidelines', *Australian Psychiatry*, 9(4), 340–44.

Meltzer, H., B. Gill and M. Petticrew (1996) *Economic Activity, Social Functioning of Residents with Psychiatric Disorders*, OCPS Surveys of Psychiatric Morbidity in Great Britain Report no. 6, London: HMSO.

Mencken, H. L. (1949) *A Mencken Chrestomathy*, New York: Vintage, 374–5.

Menon, S. (2002) 'Towards a model of psychological health empowerment; implications for health care in multicultural communities', *Nurse Education Today*, 22, 28–39.

Mental Health Commission (2004) *Quality in mental health, your views: Report on stakeholder consultation in quality in mental health services*, Dublin: Mental Health Commission.

Merleau-Ponty, M. (1962) *The Phenomenology of Perception*, tr. C. Smith, London: Routledge and Kegan Paul.

Meyer, G. and J. W. Dearing, (1996) 'Respecifying the social marketing model for unique populations', *Social Marketing Quarterly*, 3(1), 44–52.

Meyer, J. M. (2001) 'Effects of atypical antipsychotics on weight and serum lipid levels', *Journal of Clinical Psychiatry*, 62(27), 27–34.

Milio, N. (1981) *Promoting Health through Public Policy*, Philadelphia: F. A. Davis.

Milio, N. (1986) 'Promoting health through public policy' in *Introduction to Health: Policy, Planning and Financing*, ed. B. Abel-Smith, Harlow: Longman.

Millar, B. (1996) 'Creating consensus about nursing outcomes: an exploration of focus group methodology', *Journal of Clinical Nursing*, 5(4), 263–7.

Minkler, M. (1990) 'Improving health through community organisation' in *Health Education and Health Behaviour: Theory, Research and Practice*, eds. B. Reimer, F. Lewis and K. Glanz, San Francisco: Jossey-Bass.

Minkler, M. (1999) 'Personal responsibility for health? A review of the arguments and the evidence at century's end', *Health Education and Behaviour*, 26(1), 121–40.

Mitchinson, S. (1996) 'A review of the health promotion and health beliefs of traditional and project 2000 student nurses', *Journal of Advanced Nursing*, 22(1), 356–63.

Moos, R. H. and J. A. Schaefer (1987) 'Evaluating health care work settings: a holistic conceptual framework', *Psychology and Health*, 1, 97–122.

Morgan, D. (1993) *Successful Focus Groups: Advancing the State of the Art*, Newbury Park, CA: Sage.

Morgan, D. L. (1988) *Focus Groups as Qualitative Research*, Sage University Paper Series on Qualitative Research Methods, Vol. 16, Beverley Hills, USA: Sage.

Morgan, I. S. and G. W. Marsh (1998) 'Historic and future health promotion contexts for nursing', *Journal of Nursing Scholarship*, 30(4), 379–90.

Morse, J. M. and P. A. Field (1996) *Nursing Research: The Application of Qualitative Approaches*, 2nd edn, UK: Stanley Thornes Ltd.

Moser, C. A. and G. Kalton (1985) *Survey Methods in Social Investigation*, 2nd edn, Aldershot: Gower.

Murphy, L. R. (1998) 'Workplace interventions for stress reduction and prevention' in *Causes, Coping and Consequences of Stress at Work*, eds. C. L. Cooper and R. Payne, Chichester: John Wiley and Sons, 310–39.

Murphy, N., S. Jackson and M. Cronin (2005) *Annual report of Sexually Transmitted Infections 2003*, Dublin: The Health Protection Surveillance Centre.

Murphy, S. and P. Bennett (2004) 'Psychology and health promotion' in *Health Promotion: Disciplines, Diversity and Developments*, 2nd edn, eds. R. Bunton and G. Macdonald, London: Routledge.

Murray, C. J. L. and A. D. Lopez (1996) *The Global Burden of Disease*, Geneva: World Health Organization and Harvard University Press.

Mykhalovskiy, E. and L. Weir (2004) 'The problem of evidence based medicine; directions for social science', *Social Science and Medicine*, 55(5), 1059–69.

Nachmias D. and C. Frankfort-Nachmias (1992) *Research Methods in the Social Sciences*, 4th edn, New York: St Martin Press.

Nagle A., M. Schofeld and S. Redman (1999) 'Australian nurses' smoking behaviour, knowledge and attitude towards providing smoking cessation care to their patients', *Health Promotion International*, 14, 133–44.

Naidoo, J. and J. Wills (2000) *Health Promotion: Foundations for Practice*, 2nd edn, London: Balliere Tindall.

National Advisory Committee on Drugs / Drugs and Alcohol Information and Research Unit (2003) *Drug Use in Ireland and Northern Ireland: First Results from 2002–2003*, Dublin: NACD.

National Economic and Social Council (1983) *Economic and Social Policy, 1982: Aims and Recommendations*, Dublin: NESC.

National Economic and Social Council (1981) *Economic and Social Policy 1981: Aims and Recommendations*, Dublin: NESC.

National Suicide Review Group (2001) *Annual Report: Suicide Prevention across the Regions*, Galway: National Suicide Review Group.

National Taskforce on Obesity (2005) *Obesity, the Policy Challenges: The Report of the National Taskforce on Obesity*, Dublin: National Taskforce on Obesity.

Newman Giger, J. and R. E. Davidhizar, (2004) *Transcultural Nursing: Assessment and Intervention*, 4th edn, St Louis: Mosby.

Nightingale, F. (1859) *Notes on Nursing*, London: Harrison and Son.

Nolan, B. (1990) 'Socio-economic mortality differentials in Ireland', *Economic and Social Review*, 21, 193–208.

North Western Health Board (2000) *Into the Millennium and Beyond: A Strategy for Mental Health in the North West*, Leitrim: North Western Health Board.

Nutbeam, D. (1998) 'Evaluating health promotion – progress, problems and solutions', *Health Promotion International*, 3(1), 27–44.

Nutbeam, D. and E. Harris (2004) *Theory in a Nutshell: A Practical Guide to Health Promotion Theories*, Sydney: McGraw Hill.

O Donnell, K. and M. Cronin (2005) *AIDS Cases and Deaths Among AIDS Cases: Reported to end of 2004*, Dublin: The Health Protection Surveillance Centre.

OECD (2003) [Available at http://www.oecd.org/dataoecd/44/18/35044277.xls]

OECD (2005a) *Employment Outlook*, Geneva: OECD.

OECD (2005b) [Available at http://www.oecd.org/dataoecd/34/62/35027628.xls]

OECD (2005c) [Available at http://www.oecd.org/dataoecd/35/19/35027658.xls]

OECD (2005d) [Available at http://www.oecd.org/dataoecd/14/43/35029236.xls]

OECD (2005e) [Available at http://www.oecd.org/dataoecd/14/41/35029323.xls]

OECD (2005f) [Available at http://www.oecd.org/dataoecd/35/17/35027679.xls]

OECD (2005g) [Available at http://www.oecd.org/dataoecd/35/15/35027700.xls]

Office for Social Inclusion (2003) *National Action Plan against Poverty and Social Exclusion, 2003–2005*, Dublin: Department of Social and Family Affairs.

Orme, J. (2001) 'Overview of health promotion in the workplace' in *Health Promotion: Professional Perspectives*, 2nd edn, eds. A. Scriven and J. Orme, Basingstoke: Palgrave/Open University.

Ottawa Charter, *see* World Health Organization *et al.* (1986).

Papandopoulos, I. (1999) 'Health and illness beliefs of Greek Cypriots living in London', *Journal of Advanced Nursing*, 29(5), 1097–1104.

Parahoo, K. (1997) *Nursing Research: Principles, Process and Issues*, Basingstoke: Macmillan.

Park Dorsay, J. and C. Forchuk (1994) 'Assessments of the psychiatric needs of individuals with disability', *Journal of Psychiatric and Mental Health Nursing*, 1(2), 93–97.

Patton, D., K. Kolasa, S. West and T. Irons (1995) 'Sexual abstinence counselling of adolescents by physicians', *Adolescence*, 30, 963–9.

Pearsall, J., ed. (1999) *The Concise Oxford Dictionary*, 10th edn, Oxford: Oxford University Press.

Pearson, A., B. Vaughan and M. Fitzgerald (1996) *Nursing Models for Practice*, 2nd edn, Oxford: Butterworth–Heinemann.

Peplau, H. E. (1994) 'Psychiatric and mental health nursing: challenge and change', *Journal of Psychiatric and Mental Health Nursing*, 1(1), 3–7.

Phelan, M., L. Stradins and S. Morrison (2001) 'Physical health of people with severe mental illness', *British Medical Journal*, 322, 443–4.

Phillips, D. (1990) 'Postpositivistic science myths and realities' in *The Paradigm Dialogue*, ed. E. Guba, London: Sage, 31–45.

Physical Activity Group (1997) *Promoting Increased Physical Activity: A Strategy for Health Boards in Ireland*, [No publication details available].

Physical Activity Group (2001) *Promoting Increased Physical Activity: A Review of the National Strategy for Health Boards 1997–2000*, Dublin: The Office for Health Gain.

Piper, S. M. and P. A. Brown (1998) 'The theory and practice of health education applied to nursing: a bipolar approach', *Journal of Advanced Nursing*, 27(2), 383–9.

Plant, R. (2003) 'Citizenship and social society', *Fiscal Studies*, 2(2), 153–66.

Pocock, B. (2001) *The Effect of Long Hours on Family and Community Life*, A report for the Queensland Department of Industrial Relations.

Polit, D. F. and B. P. Hungler (1995) *Nursing Research: Principles and Methods*, Philedelphia: Lippincott.

Polit, D. F., C. T. Beck and B. P. Hungler (1999) *Nursing Research: Principles and Methods*, 6th edn, Philadelphia: Lippincott.

Powell, J. (1999) 'Monitoring and evaluation in cardiac rehabilitation' in *Evidenced Based Health Promotion*, eds. E. R. Perkins, I. Simnet and L. Wright, Chichester: John Wiley and sons, 377–85.

Prescott, E., P. Lange and J. Vestbo (1999) 'Socioeconomic status, lung function and admission to hospital for COPD: results from the Copenhagen City Heart Study', *European Respiratory Journal*, 13(5), 1109–14.

Prospectus Report, *see* Government of Ireland (2003a).

Prior, J. O., G. Van Melle, A. Crisinel, B. Burnand, J. Cornuz and R. Darioli (2005) 'Evaluation of a multicomponent worksite health promotion program for cardiovascular risk factors – correcting for the regression towards the mean effect', *Preventive Medicine*, 40, 259–67.

Prochaska, J. O. (1979) *Systems of Psychotherapy: A Transtheoretical Analysis*, Homewood, IL: Dorsey Press.

Prochaska, J. O. and C. C. DiClemente (1983) 'Stages and processes of self–change of smoking: toward an integrative model of change', *Journal of Counseling and Clinical Psychology*, 51, 390–5.

Prochaska, J. O. and C. C. DiClemente (1984) *The Transtheoretical Approach: Crossing Traditional Boundaries of Therapy*, Homewood, IL: Dow Jones Irwin.

Prochaska, J. O. and C. C. DiClemente (1986) 'Toward a comprehensive model of change' in *Treating Addictive Behaviours: Processes of Change*, eds. W. Miller and N. Heather, New York: Plenum Press.

Prochaska, J. O., C. C. DiClemente and J. C. Norcross (1992) 'In search of how people change', *American Psychologist*, 47, 1102–14.

Punch, K. (1998) *Introduction to Social Research, Quantitative and Qualitative Approaches*, London: Sage.

Putnam, R. (1993) *Making Democracy Work*, New Jersey: Princeton University Press.

Putnam, R. (1995) 'Bowling alone, America's declining social capital', *Journal of Democracy*, 6, 65–78.

Ramos, M. C. (1992) 'The nurse–patient relationship: theme and variations', *Journal of Advanced Nursing*, 17(4), 469–506.

Ramstedt, M. and A. Hope (2005) 'The Irish drinking habits of 2002: drinking and drinking-related harm, a European comparative perspective', *Journal of Substance Use*, 10(5), 273–383(11).

Rappaport, J., C. Swift and R. Hess (1984) *Studies in Empowerment: Steps toward Understanding and Action*, New York: Haworth.

Rasmussen, V. and D. Rivett (2000) 'The European network of health promoting schools – an alliance of health, education and democracy', *Health Education*, 100(2), 61–7.

Rehn, N., R. Room and G. Edwards (2001) *Alcohol in the European Region: Consumption, Harm and Policies*, Copenhagen: World Health Organization Regional office for Europe.

Reid, A. and J. Malone (2003) 'A cross-sectional study of needs and priorities within the Irish civil service', *Occupational Medicine*, 53, 41–5.

Rissel, C., L. McLellan and A. Bauman (2000) 'Social factors associated with ethnic differences in alcohol and marijuana use in Vietnamese, Arabic and English-speaking youths in Sydney, Australia', *Journal of Paediatric Child Health*, 36, 145–52.

Roberts, P. (1997) 'Planning and running a focus group: qualitative data analysis', *Nurse Researcher*, 4(4), 79.

Robinson, N. (1999) 'The use of focus group methodology – with selected examples from sexual health research', *Journal of Advanced Nursing*, 29, 905–13.

Rodin, J. and P. Salovey (1989) 'Health psychology', *Annual Review of Psychology*, 40, 533–79.

Rogers, E. (1983) *Diffusion of Innovations*, 3rd edn, New York: Free Press.

Ronayne, A. (2001) 'Nurse–patient partnerships in hospital care', editorial, *Journal of Clinical Nursing*, 10(5), 591–2.

Rosenstock, L. (1966) 'Why people use health services', *Millbank Memorial Fund Quarterly*, 44, 94–124.

Rosenstock, L. (1974) 'Historical origins of the health belief model', *Health Education Monographs*, 2, 1–8.

Rowe, K. and J. Macleod Clark (1999) 'Evaluating the effectiveness of a smoking cessation intervention designed for nurses', *International Journal of Nursing Studies*, 36(4), 301–11.

Rowe, K. and J. Macleod Clark (2000), 'The incidence of smoking amongst nurses: a review of the literature', *Journal of Advanced Nursing*, 31(5), 1046–53.

Royal College of Nursing (1996) *Sexual Health: Key Issues within Mental Health Services*, London: Royal College of Nursing.

Rumbold, G. (2000) *Ethics in Nursing Practice*, 3rd edn, London: Balliere Tindall.

Rush, K. L., C. C. Kee and M. Rice (2005) 'Nurses as imperfect role models for health promotion', *Western Journal of Nursing Research*, 27(2), 166–83.

Ryan, D. (2003a) 'Indicators of work stress among Irish public service employees', unpublished doctoral thesis, University College Cork.

Ryan, D. (2003b) 'The person who is paranoid or suspicious' in *Psychiatric and Mental Health Nursing: The Craft of Caring*, ed. P. Barker, London: Arnold, 305–11.

Ryan, D. and E. Quayle (1999) 'Stress in psychiatric nursing – fact or fiction', *Nursing Standard*, 14(8), 32–5.

Rycroft-Malone, J., G. Harvey, K. Seers, A. Kitson, B. McCormack and A. Titchen (2004) 'An exploration of the factors that influence the implementation of evidence into practice', *Journal of Clinical Nursing*, 13, 913–24.

Sackett, D. L., W. M. C. Rosenberg, J. A. Muir Gray, R. B. Haynes and W. S. Richardson (1996) 'Evidence based medicine: what it is and what it isn't', *British Journal of Medicine*, 312, 71–2.

Sackett, D., S. Straus, W. Richardson, W. Rosenberg and R. Hynes (2000) *Evidence Based Medicine: How to Practice and Teach EBM*, 2nd edn, Edinburgh: Churchill Livingstone.

Sadala, M. L. A. and R. de Camargo Ferreira Adorno (2002) 'Phenomenology as a method to investigate the experience lived: a perspective from Husserl and Merleau-Ponty's thought', *Journal of Advanced Nursing*, 37(3), 282–93.

Sanders, D., V. Stone, G. Fowler and J. Marziller (1986) 'Practice, nurses and anti-smoking legislation', *British Medical Journal*, 292, 381–3.

SANE Australia (2000) *The Sane Smoke Free Kit*, Melbourne: SANE Australia.

Sarafino, E. P. (1998) *Health Psychology: Biopsychosocial Interactions*, 3rd edn, New York: Wiley and Sons.

Sarason S. (1996) *Barometers of Change: Individual, Educational and Social Transformation*, San Francisco: Jossey-Bass.

Sarna, L. (1999) 'Hope and vision prevention: tobacco control and cancer nursing', *Cancer Nursing*, 22(1), 21–8.

Scarinci, I. C., B. M. Beech, W. Naumann, K. W. Kovach, L. Pugh and B. Fapohunda (2002) 'Depression, socioeconomic status, age, and marital status in black women: a national study', *Ethnicity and Disease*, 12(3), 421–8.

Schein, E. H. (1987), *Process Consultation*, II: *Lessons for Managers and Consultants*, Reading, MA: Addison-Wesley.

Schein, E. (1985) *Organisational Culture and Leadership*, San Francisco: Jossey-Bass.

Senior, B. (1997) *Organisational Change*, London: Pitman.

Simons-Morton, B. G., W. H. Green and N. H. Gottlieb (1995) *Introduction to Health Education and Health Promotion*, 2nd edn, Prospect Heights, IL: Waveland.

Sines, D. (1994) 'The arrogance of power: a reflection on contemporary mental health nursing practice', *Journal of Advanced Nursing*, 20(5), 894–903.

Soeken, K. L., R. B. Bausell and M. Winklestein (1989) 'Preventative behaviour: attitudes and compliance of nursing students', *Journal of Advanced Nursing*, 14(12), 1026–33.

Sourtzi, P., P. Nolan and R. Andrews (1996) 'Evaluation of health promotion activities in community nursing practice', *Journal of Advanced Nursing*, 24, 1214–23.

Spielberg, H. (1960) *The Phenomenological Movement: A Historical Introduction*, 2nd edn, 2 vols., The Hague: Nijhoff.

Spring, B., R. Pingitore and D. E. McChargue (2003) 'Reward value of cigarette smoking for comparably heavy smoking schizophrenic, depressed and non-smoking patients', *American Journal of Psychiatry*, 160(2), 316–22.

Sports Council / Health Education Authority (1992) *Allied Dunbar National Fitness Survey*, London: Sports Council / Health Education Authority.

Stenhouse, L. (1975) *An Introduction to Curriculum Research and Development*, London: Heinemann.

Stenhouse, L. (1985) 'What counts as research?' in *Research as a Basis for Teaching*, eds. J. Ruddock and D. Hopkins, London: Heinemann.

Steptoe, A., S. Doherty, T. Kendrick, E. Rink and S. Hilton (1999) 'Attitudes to cardiovascular health promotion among GPs and practice nurses', *Family Practice*, 16, 158–63.

Stevens, P. E. (1996) 'Focus groups: collecting aggregate-level data to understand community health phenomena', *Public Health Nursing*, 13, 170–6.

Stewart, D. W. and P. N. Shamdasani (1990) *Focus Groups: Theory and Practice*, Newbury Park: Sage.

Stone, G. L., P. Jebsen, P. Walk and R. Belsham (1984) 'Identification of stress and coping skills within a critical care setting', *Western Journal of Nursing Research*, 6, 201–11.

Strauss, A. and J. Corbin (1990) *Basics of Qualitative Research: Techniques and Procedures for Developing Grounded Theory*, Thousand Oaks: Sage.

Svedberg. P., H. Jormfeldt and B. Arvidsson (2003) 'Patients' conceptions of how health processes are promoted in mental health nursing: a qualitative study', *Journal of Advanced Nursing*, 10(4), 448–52.

Taylor, L. (1998a) 'Mental health promotion in Canada: working towards a national plan of action for promoting the mental health of Canadians', paper presented at the Clifford Beers Conference, Birmingham.

Taylor, M., D. Ryan, E. Quayle and K. O'Sullivan (1998b) *Stress and Coping Among Members of the Garda Siochána*, Cork: Department of Applied Psychology, University College Cork.

Taylor, M. A. (1998c) 'Evidence based practice: are dieticians willing and able?', *Journal of Human Nutrition and Dietetics*, 11, 461–72.

Than, M., S. Bidwell, C. Davison, R. Phibbs and M. Walker (2005) 'Evidence based emergency at the "coal face"', *Emergency Medicine Australasia*, 17, 330–40.

Thomas, S. P. (2005) 'Through the lens of Merleau-Ponty: advancing the phenomenological approach to nursing research', *Nursing Philosophy*, 6, 63–76.

Thorogood, N. (2004) 'What is the relevance of sociology for health promotion?' in *Health Promotion: Disciplines, Diversity and Developments*, 2nd edn, eds. R. Bunton and G. Macdonald, London: Routledge.

Thornthwaite, L. (2002) *Work-family Balance: International Research on Employee Preferences*, Sydney: ACIRRT, University of Sydney, 8.

Todd, C. (2004) *Improving Work Life Balance, What Are Other Countries Doing?*, Canada: Labour Program Human Resources and Skills Development.

Tones, K. (1990) 'Why theorise? Ideology in health promotion', *Health Education Journal*, 49(1), 2–6.

Tones, K. and G. Green (2004) *Health Promotion: Planning and Strategies*, London: Sage.

Torre, D. (1986) *Empowerment: Structured Conceptualisation and Instrument*, New York: Cornell University.

Townsend, P., N. Davidson and M. Whitehead (1988) *Inequalities in Health, the Black Report and the Health Divide*, London: Penguin.

Underwood, P. W. (1998) 'Breast cancer awareness begins with you', *American Journal of Nursing*, 98(10), 80.

United Nations (1948) [Available at http:www.un.org/overview/rights.html]

Upshur, R. E. G. (2000) 'Seven characteristics of medical evidence', *Journal of Evaluation in Clinical Practice*, 6(2), 93–7.

Usher, P. (1996) 'Feminist approaches to research' in *Understanding Educational Research*, eds. D. Scott and R. Usher, London: Routledge.

Van Dongen, C. J. and K. A. Fox (1999) 'Smoking and persistent mental illness: an exploratory study', *Journal of Psychosocial Nursing*, 37(11), 26–34.

Waar, P. (1990) 'The measurement of wellbeing and other aspects of mental health', *Journal of Occupational Psychology*, 63, 193–210.

Wai, C-T., M-L. Wong, S. Ng, A. Cheok, M-H. Tan, W. Chua, B. Mak, M-O. Aung and S-G. Lim (2005) 'Utility of the health belief model in predicting compliance of screening in patients with chronic hepatitis B', *Alimentary Pharmacology and Therapeutics*, 21(10) 1255–62.

Walker, K. (2003) 'Why evidence based practice now?: a polemic', *Nursing Inquiry*, 10, 145–55.

Wall, K. and J. São José (2004) 'Managing work and care: a difficult challenge for immigrant families', *Social Policy and Administration*, 38(6), 591–621.

Wallace, B. and C. Tennant (1998) 'Nutrition and obesity in the chronic mentally ill', *Australian and New Zealand Journal of Psychiatry*, 32(1), 82–5.

Wallerstein, N. (1992) 'Powerlessness, empowerment and health: implications from health promotion programmes', *American Journal of Health Promotion*, 6(3), 197–205.

Warr, P. (1994) 'A conceptual framework for the study of work and mental health', *Work and Stress*, 8(2), 84–97.

Warr, P. B. (1987) *Work, Unemployment, and Mental Health*, Oxford: Oxford University Press.

Webb, C. (1999) 'Analysing qualitative data: computerised and other approaches', *Journal of Advanced Nursing*, 29(2), 323–30.

Wells, J. S. G., D. Ryan, C. N. McElwee, M. Boyce and C. J. Forkan (2000) *Worthy Not Worthwhile? Choosing Careers in Caring Occupations*, Waterford: Centre for Social Care Research, Waterford Institute of Technology.

Weinhardt, L. S., M. P. Carey and K. B. Carey (1997) 'HIV risk education for the seriously mentally ill. Pilot investigation and call for research', *Journal of Behavioural Therapy and Experimental Psychiatry*, 28, 87–95.

Weisberg, H. E., J. A. Krosnick and B. D. Bowen (1996) *An Introduction to Survey Research, Polling and Data Analysis*, 3rd edn, Thousand Oaks: Sage.

Wewers, M. E., K. L. Ahijevych and L. Sarna (1998) 'Smoking cessation interventions in nursing practice', *Nursing Clinics of North America*, 33(1), 61–74.

Whitehead, D. (2001) 'Health education, behavioural change and social psychology: nursing's contribution to health promotion', *Journal of Advanced Nursing*, 34(6), 310–21.

Whitehead, D. (2003) 'Evaluating health promotion: a model for nursing practice', *Journal of Advanced Nursing*, 41(5), 490–98.

Whitehead, D. (2004) 'Health promotion and health education: advancing the concepts', *Journal of Advanced Nursing*, 47(3), 311–20.

Whitehead, J. (1989) 'Creating a living educational theory from questions of the kind "How do I improve my practice?"', *Cambridge Journal of Education*, 19(1), 41–52.

Whitmer, R. (1993) 'Why we should foster health promotion?', *Business and Health*, 11(13), 74–6.

WHO (1946) *Constitution*, Geneva: WHO.

WHO (1978) *Report of the Primary Health Care Conference: Alma Ata*, Geneva: WHO.

WHO (1984) *Health Promotion: A Discussion Document on the Concepts and the Principles*, Copenhagen: WHO.

WHO (1986) *The Ottawa Charter for Health Promotion*, Ottawa: Canadian Public Health Association.

WHO (1988) *The Adelaide Recommendations, Healthy Public Policy*, Copenhagen: WHO/EURO.

WHO (1991) *Sundsvall Statement on Supportive Environments for Health*, Geneva: WHO.

WHO (1993) *Life Skills Education in Schools*, Geneva: WHO.

WHO (1994) *Declaration on Occupational Health for All*, Geneva: WHO.

WHO (1997) *The Jakarta Declaration on Leading Health Promotion into the 21st Century*, Geneva: WHO.

WHO (1998) *Health for All in the 21st Century*, European Health for All Series, no. 5, Copenhagen: WHO.

WHO (1998) *Health Promotion Glossary*, Geneva: WHO.

WHO (2000) *Health Promotion: Bridging the Equity Gap*, Mexico: WHO.

WHO (2001a) *World Health Report*, Geneva: WHO.

WHO (2001b) *The World Health Report 2001: Mental Health – New Understanding, New Hope*, Geneva: WHO.

WHO (2002a) *The European Health Report*, European Series, no. 97, Copenhagen: WHO Regional Publications.

WHO (2002b) *The World Health Report: Reducing Risks, Promoting Healthy life*, Geneva: WHO.

Wiley, M. M. (1997) 'Hospital financing in selected member states of the European Union' in *Health Care and its Financing in the Single European Market*, ed. R. Leidl, Biomedical and Health Research Series, Volume 18, Amsterdam: IOS Press.

Wiley, M. M. (1998) 'Health expenditure trends in Ireland: past, present and future' in *The Irish Health System in the 21st Century*, eds. A. L. Leahy and M. M. Wiley, Dublin: Oak Tree Press.

Wilkinson, R. (1996) *Unequal Societies: The Affliction of Inequality*, London: Routledge.

Williams, A. (1993) 'Community health learning experiences and political activism: a model for baccalaureate curriculum revolution content', *Journal of Nursing Education*, 32(8), 352–6.

Wilson, G. (1993) *Making Change Happen*, London: Pitman.

Wilson-Barnett, J. and S. Latter (1993) 'Factors influencing nurses' health education and health promotion practice in acute ward areas', in *Research in Health Promotion and Nursing*, eds. J. Wilson-Barnett and J. Macleod Clark, London: Macmillan.

Winch, S., D. Creedy and W. Chaboyer (2002) 'Governing nursing conduct: the rise of evidence based practice', *Nursing Inquiry*, 9(3), 156–61.

Winter, R. and C. Munn-Giddings (2001) *A Handbook for Action Research in Health and Social Care*, London: Routledge.

Woodrow, P. (1997) 'Nurse advocacy: is it in the patient's best interests?', *British Journal of Nursing*, 6(4), 225–9.

World Medical Association (1964, 2000) *World Medical Association Declaration of Helsinki: Ethical Principles for Medical Research Involving Human Subjects*. [Available at <http://www.wma.net/e/policy/b3.htm]

Wren, B. and K. Thomas (2001) *Brief Intervention Skills for Health Promotion*, Dublin: Health Promotion Department.

Wynne, R. (1993) 'Action for health at work: the next steps', policy paper, Dublin: European Foundation for the Improvement of Living and Working Conditions.

Wynne, R. (1995) *A Training Specification for Workplace Health Promotion*, Dublin: Work Research Centre.

Xiao, J. J., B. O'Neill, J. M. Prochaska, C. M. Kerbel, P. Brennan and B. J. Bristow (2004) 'A consumer education programme based on the transtheoretical model of change', *International Journal of Consumer Studies*, 28(1), 55–6.

Yuro-Petro, H. and B. R. Scanelli (1992) 'The education of health care professionals in the year 2000 and beyond: Part 1: a consumers view', *Health Care Supervisor*, 10(3), 1–11.

Index

absenteeism, 61, 64, 70, 71
accountability, 17, 105
action, theory of reasoned action, 37
action research, 47, 126–32
    model of, 127
Adolescent Health Strategy, 90
adoptive leave, 64
advocacy, 15
    community empowerment, 53, 54
    grounded theory and, 123, 125
    nurses' role, 82
Age and Opportunity, 58
AIDS, 60, 98
Ajzen, I. and Fishbein, M., 37
alcohol consumption, 19, 59
    binge drinking, 59
    statistics, 26, 59
Allied Dunbar Fitness Survey, 57
Alma Ata Declaration, 12
Amnesty International, 96, 100
anonymity, right to, 144–5, 154, 156, 160
Anthony, P. and Crawford, P., 83
Asclepius, 1–2
assertiveness training, 51
assessment *see* evaluation
assessment of needs, 45
asylum seekers, 92
attentiveness, 119
autonomy, respect for, 141–2
Aware, 88
axial coding, 163

backward mapping, 45
Baird, C., 161
Bandura, A., 35, 40–1, 44, 51, 75, 84
Barker, D. and Rose, G., 7
Baum, F. and Palmer, C., 53
Baum, F. and Ziersch, A., 53
Beauchamp, T. and Childress, J., 140
behaviour, 36 *see also* individual change
Being Well programme, 58
beneficence, 140
Benner, P. and Tanner, C., 118
Bennett, N., Glatter, R. and Levacic, R., 156
Benson, A. and Latter, S., 81
best practice, 103
Better Health through Prevention, 19

Bhugra, D., 93
Bí Folláin, 77
biomedical model of health, 2, 4–5, 16
    expert power, 50–1
    nurses' role, 80, 83
    reductionism, 84, 87–8, 106
    research evidence, 105–6
    scientific knowledge, 109
Black Report (1980), 10
Bodywhys, 88
Bord Altranais, An, 79, 89
Bourdieu, Pierre, 114
bracketing, 112, 119, 120, 121
brainstorming, 160–1
Brennan, D., 5, 88
Brennan Report (2003), 28
Brentano, Franz, 116–17
brief interventions model of change, 42, 80–1
Brief Interventions Skills for Health Promotion
        programme, 42
British Dietetic Association, 104
Brown, R. and Adebayo, S., 62
Brown, S. *et al.*, 96
Buchanan, C. *et al.*, 97
bureaucracy, 67

Callaghan, P., 99
capacity building, 53–4, 81, 86
Caplan, A., 139
cardiovascular diseases, 65, 72, 96
cardiovascular strategy, 19
carers' groups, 54
Carey, P., 49
Carper, B., 105
Carr, W. and Kemmis, S., 126, 127
Cartesian dualism, 84–5, 118
Cataldo, J., 97
census, population, 165, 166
Centre for Health Promotion Studies (CHPS), 10,
    58
change management, 34–47, 75
    brief interventions model, 42, 80–1
    change agents, 44–7
    defining change, 34–5
    diffusion of innovations theory, 44
    force field analysis, 43
    health belief model, 36–7

change management, *continued*
   individual change, 35–42, 55
   Lewin's unfreezing/freezing model, 42–3
   organisational change, 42–7
   social cognition theory, 40–2, 44, 75
   stages of change model, 37–40, 75, 80
   theory of reasoned action, 37
Charting our Education Future, 77
citizenship, 91–2
Civil Service, 71
CLAN (College Lifestyle and Attitudinal
      National) survey, 58, 59, 90
Cobban, S., 107
Cochrane, A., 103
Code of Professional Conduct (An Bord
      Altranais), 79
codes of practice, 139, 144
coding (data analysis), 163, 171
Cohen, L., Manion, L. and Morrison, K., 151
Cohen, M., 116, 117, 118
Colaizzi, P., 121
collectivism, 6, 22
Commission of Inquiry on Mental Handicap, 28
Commission of Inquiry on Mental Illness, 28
commonality of purpose, 67
communication theory, 75
communities, 53
   capacity building, 53–4, 81
   change theory, 44
   definition of, 53
   empowerment, 53–4, 81
         in Ireland, 54
community care, 11
   programme expenditures, 27
Community Mothers Programme, 87
competence to consent, 143
'completeness', 2 *see also* holistic concept of
      health
confidentiality, 142, 143, 155, 160
   right to, 144–5
consciousness, intentionality of, 117–18
consent, 142
   competence and, 143
   free choice and, 143
   informed, 142, 154, 176
constant-comparison model, 125
constructivism, 111–12, 117, 120, 121
   grounded theory, 124
consumer movement, 104
contingency planning, 29
control groups, 135
convenience sampling, 168
Cool School programme, 87
Cooper, C. *et al.*, 68

Cort, E. *et al.*, 98
Côté-Arsenault, D. and Morrisson-Beedy, D.,
      157
Cox, E., 53
Cox, T. and Ferguson, E., 67
Crehan, M., 99
Creswell, J., 173
critical reflection, 134–5
critical theory, 113–15, 126
cues to action, 36
culture, 91–6
   defining, 93
   health factors and, 9, 10, 55, 56
   health promotion, 91–6
   Travelling community, 94–6
culture of organisations, 68–70

Dahlgren, G. and Whitehead, M., 7–8
data analysis, 163–4, 171–2
   coding, 163, 171
   descriptive/inferential, 171–2
   focus groups, 163–4
   funnelling, 163
   phenomenology, 121–2
   software packages, 175
   surveys, 171–2
data collection, 137, 165–6
   action research, 128, 130
   focus groups, 157–8
   grounded theory, 124–5
   surveys, 166–71
data protection, 143
databases, 149
Davidson, S. *et al.*, 96, 98
Deasy, C., 79, 84, 98
death rates *see* mortality rates
deontological philosophy, 140
depression, 65, 85, 86, 87, 89, 97
Dept of Education and Science, 77
Dept of Health and Children, 9–10, 17, 30, 77,
      81, 82, 88
Dept of Local Government and Public Health, 25
Descartes, René, 2, 84–5
determinants of health, 6–9, 55, 56
diet and nutrition, 60
dieticians, 17
diffusion of innovations theory, 44
dignity, 142–3
disclosure, right to, 142, 143, 144, 145
discrimination, 64, 86
disease
   concept of, 2
   disease prevention, 28, 30
   'handling disease' concept, 23

see also illness
disempowerment, 50, 113–15 *see also* empowerment
dispensary system, 24
double effect, principle of, 141
Downie, R., Tannahill, C. and Tannahill, A., 10–11
drinking *see* alcohol consumption
drug abuse, 59–60, 77
  statistics, 59
dualism, Cartesian, 84–5, 118
Duasco, M. and Cheung, P., 79
Duxbury, L. and Higgins, C., 61

early adopters of change, 44
Early School Leaving Project, 54
eating patterns, 60
education, health promotion in, 75–8
  curriculum provision, 77
  experiential learning cycle, 76–7
  initiatives, 78
    Irish, 76, 77, 87
Education Act 1998, 77
Education and Science, Dept of, 77
effect, principle of double effect, 141
elitism, 113, 114
Elliott, J., 127
Elmore, R., 45
emancipation, 113–15
'emic' position, 112
empirical research, 105, 110–11, 123
employment *see* work
Employment Discrimination Act 1998, 64
empowerment, 14–15, 48–54
  action research and, 126, 131
  community development, 53–4
  concept and definition, 48–9, 52
  critical theory and, 113–15
  Irish context, 18, 54
  nurses' role, 78, 79
  of nurses, 81–3
  power concept, 14, 50–2
    types of power, 50
  practitioner–client relationship, 49, 50–2
  social capital and, 52–3
ENHPS (European Network of Health-Promoting Schools), 78
enslavement, 113
environment, as health determinant, 7–9, 10, 41, 55, 56
epidemiology, 7, 8, 106
Equal Status Act 2000, 94
Equality Working Group, 54
equity, 13, 14, 17, 18

critical theory, 113–15
ethics, 139–45
  action research and, 131
  autonomy, respect for, 141–2
  beneficence, 140
  in focus groups, 160
  justice principle, 142
  non-maleficence, 141
  proposed research, 176
  protection function, 139–42
  protocols, 176
  research contracts, 144
  rights of human beings, 142–5
ethnicity
  health factors and, 9, 10, 55, 56
  health promotion, 91–6
'etic' position, 110
European Foundation for the Improvement of Living and Working Conditions, 64
European Network for Workplace Health Promotion, 70
European Network of Health-Promoting Schools (ENHPS), 78
European Union, 28, 32–3, 91
evaluation, 133–8
  evaluating change, 46–7
  planning an evaluation, 136–8
  types of, 134–5
evidence, hierarchies of, 150
evidence-based practice, 103–7
exercise, 56–8
expenditure in health services, 24, 26
  by programme, 27
  resource agendas, 103–4
experiential learning cycle, 76–7
experiments, research, 105, 110, 119
expert power, 50–1

fairness principle, 142
  right to fair treatment, 143–4
Falk-Rafael, A., 52
Family Friendly Workplace Day, 63
Fás le Cheile, 87
feedback, 134 *see also* evaluation
feminist research, 114, 126
Fink, A. and Kosecoff, J., 166
fitness surveys, 57
focus groups, 157–64
  data analysis, 163–4
  ethical issues, 160
  planning and facilitating, 158–63
  role of facilitator, 162–3
  selecting target-group sample, 159–60
Fontaine, K., 85

force field analysis, 43
force majeure leave, 64
formative evaluation, 134
Foucault, Michel, 50–1, 114
Frankfurt School, 113, 114
free choice, right to, 143
Freire, Paulo, 49, 51, 54
French, P., 104
Fuimano, J., 62, 63

Gadamer, Hans-Georg, 120
Galen, 56, 84
Gallup, George, 165
Garda Síochána, 67
General Hospital Programme, 27
General Support Programme, 27
genetic factors, and health, 7, 9, 10, 55
Gillon, R., 141
Glaser, B., 125
   and Strauss, A., 123–4
globalisation, 27–8
Go for Life Campaign, 58
Gray, R. *et al.*, 98
grounded theory, 123–5
group interviews, 157 *see also* focus groups
Grow, 88

Habermas, J., 114
Handy, C., 68
Happy Heart at Work programme, 72
harm
   non-maleficence, 141
   right to protection from harm, 143–4
Harrison, D., 32
HBSC (Health Behaviour in School-aged
   Children), 10
health, 1–10
   concepts, 2–3
   defining, 1–5, 12–13
   determinants of health, 6–9, 55, 56
   factors influencing, 5–9
   individual choice v. collectivism, 6, 22–3
   a 'state of being', 3, 6
   WHO influence, 3–5
   work and, 61, 65–7
   work–life balance, 61–4
   see also lifestyles; public policy
Health Act 1970, 16, 25
Health and Children, Dept of, 9–10, 17, 30, 77,
   81, 82, 88
'health and social gain', 16
Health at Work programme, 72
Health Behaviour in School-aged Children
   (HBSC), 10

health belief model, 36–7
health boards, 25–6, 58
health economics, 103–4
health education, traditional, 11, 14, 76
   nurses confuse with health promotion, 79, 80,
      81
'Health for all by the year 2000', 12
health motivation, 36
Health of Our Children, 90
health promotion, 10–20
   change advocacy *see* change management
   defining, 10–13, 75
   definition (Ottawa Charter), 13
   distinct from health education, 11, 14, 76
   in education, 75–8
   ethnic groups, 91–6
   historical development, 11–13
   individual choice v. collectivism, 6, 22–3
   integration, 12
   Irish context, 9–10, 16–20, 56, 79 *see also*
      public policy
   mental health *see* mental health promotion
   nurses *see* nurses and health promotion
   politicisation, 11
   principles of, 13–15, 18
   psychology, 74–5
   'settings approach', 70
   sociology, 73–4
   in workplace, 70–2
      Ireland, 72
   see also lifestyles; public policy; research
Health Promotion Unit, 9–10
Health Service Executive, 25, 30
health services in Ireland
   aims of, 17–18
   expenditure, 24, 26
      by programme, 27
   globalisation and, 27–8
   health promotion strategy, 9–10, 16–20, 56, 79
      staff and resources, 17
   historical development, 24–6, 28, 30
   mental illness, 87, 88–91, 96–100
   planning and strategy, 21–3, 28–30
   public policy, 21–33
      'healthy public policy', 20, 23, 31–2, 74
   social policy, 23–6, 74
   see also nurses
Health, the Wider Dimension, 26
Healthy People: The Surgeon General's Report,
   12
Healthy People 2000, 12
'healthy public policy' concept, 20, 23, 31–2, 74
Heidegger, Martin, 112, 117, 118, 119, 120
Henderson, Virginia, 78

Hewinson, A., 82
Hewitt, J., 82
Hippocrates, 84, 141
HIV, 60, 98
Hjelm, K. *et al.*, 93
Hochbaum, G., 36
Hodge, M., 63
Hodgson, R., 86
holistic concept of health, 2–3, 4–5, 6–7, 13, 23, 84–5
    education and, 77
    mental health, 84–5, 88
    nurses' role, 78, 79
    phenomenology, 119
    physical activity, 56, 85
Hope, A. *et al.*, 79
Hope, P., 163
Horkheimer, M., 113, 114
Husserl, Edmund, 112, 116–17, 118, 119, 120
Hussey, D., 47
Hycner, R., 163
Hygeia, 1
Hyland, B. *et al.*, 98, 99

ideologies, definition and critique of, 114
illness
    client disempowerment, 50
    concept of, 2–3
    defining, 2
    factors leading to, 7
    'handling disease' concept, 23
    prevention, 28, 30
        health belief model, 36–7
    role of nurses, 78, 80
immigration, 92–3
individual change, 35–42, 55
    brief interventions model, 42, 80–1
    health belief model, 36–7
    motivation, 36, 40
    relapse, 40
    social cognition theory, 40–2, 44, 75
    stages of change model, 37–40, 75, 80
    theory of reasoned action, 37
individualism, 6, 22
individuality, and autonomy, 141–2
inductive approaches, 123
inequity, 14, 74, 113 *see also* equity
information
    dissemination, 176–7
    literature reviews, 146–50
    sources, primary/secondary, 148–9
information-giving, 11, 14, 75, 76, 81
informed consent, 142, 154, 176
integration, and health promotion, 12

intentionality, 67
intentionality of consciousness, 117–18
internet, information sources, 149
interpersonal factors, as health determinants, 8, 9
interpretivism, 111–12, 117, 120, 121
        grounded theory, 124
intersubjectivity, 119
interviews, 151–6
    effective, 153–6
    group interviews, 157 *see also* focus groups
    phenomenological research, 120–1, 153
    pitfalls, 156
    structured/unstructured, 152–3
intuiting, phenomenological, 117, 118
intuition, 118
Irish Heart Foundation, 58, 72

Jackson, S. *et al.*, 49
Jakarta Declaration (1997), 14, 70
Jasper, M., 119
job flexibility, 63, 64
job sharing, 64
Johnson, M., 117
Jones, A., 61, 64
Jones, L., 3, 4
justice principle, 142

Kelleher, C., 72
Kemmis, S. and Carr, W., 126, 127
Kemmis, S. and McTaggart, R., 127
knowledge
    phenomenological intuiting, 117, 118
    positivist research, 110–11
    positivist tradition, 105, 108, 109
    power and, 50–1
    scientific, 105, 108, 109
Kolb, D., 76
Krueger, R., 158, 159, 160, 161, 163
    and Casey, M., 157
Kuhn, T., 27, 109
Kunitz, S., 52
Kvale, S., 151

La Ferla, A., 67
LaLonde, M., 56
language, terminology and power, 50–1
learning
    experiential learning cycle, 76–7
    social learning theory, 40–2, 44, 75, 84
    vicarious, 41, 44
'lebenswelt', 119–20
legal accountability, 105
Lewin, Kurt, 42–3, 127
Lewis, J. and Scott, E., 98

liberation theology, 126
libraries, 149
life expectancy, 26
Lifestyle Challenge, 58
lifestyles, 55–60
    changing *see* individual change
    diet and nutrition, 60
    drug use, 59–60, 77
    as health determinants, 6, 7, 9, 55–6
    health promotion, 11, 55–6
    individual choice v. collectivism, 6, 22–3
    in Ireland, 10, 18–19
        government strategy, 56, 57–8
    mentally ill, 96–9
    of nurses, 83–4
    physical activity, 56–8
    sexual health, 60
    victim blaming, 56
    young people, 58, 59, 77
    see also alcohol consumption; smoking
Lifewise programme, 58
life-world, 118, 119–20
Limerick, Myross Community Development
    Network, 54
literature reviews, 146–50
    primary/secondary sources, 148–9
    writing research proposals, 174
litigation, 105
lived experience, 118, 119–20
living theory, 129
LoBionda-Wood, G. and Harber, J., 140
Locke, L. *et al.*, 173
locus of control, 75
Lukes, S., 52

Maben, J. and Macleod Clark, J., 79
Making the Healthier Choice the Easier Choice,
    9, 90
Mannix McNamara, P., 51
Marcel, Gabriel, 117
Marshall, C. and Rossman, G., 163
Mason, R., 49
maternity leave, 64
Maville, J. and Huerta, C., 83, 99
McAuliffe, E. and Joyce, L., 30
McCubbin, M., 48, 50
McKevitt, D., 30
McKinsey and Company, 25
McNamara, C., 67
McNiff, J., 126, 130
meaning, and phenomenology, 116
medicine, traditional model, 2, 4–5, 16
    expert power, 50–1
    nurses' role, 80, 83

reductionism, 84, 87–8, 106
research evidence, 105–6
scientific knowledge, 105, 108, 109
Mencken, H.L., 3
Mental Health Commission, 99, 100
Mental Health into the Millennium and Beyond,
    90
Mental Health Ireland, 87, 88
Mental Health Matters, 87
mental health promotion, 84–91
    aims and strategies, 86–7
    defining, 86
    defining mental health, 84–5
    services and responsibility, 87–91
        Irish, 87, 88–91
    see also mental illness
*Mental Health Promotion: A Quality
    Framework*, 85
Mental Hospitals Report (2001), 96
mental illness, 96–100
    defining, 85
    lifestyles, 96–9
    nurses' role, 79, 80, 83
    physical illness link, 88, 96
    psychiatric nursing objectives, 89
    reports, 28, 88, 90, 96
    rights and access to services, 96
    sexuality and, 98–9
    smoking and, 97–8
    stigma, 99–100
    see also mental health promotion
Merleau-Ponty, Maurice, 117, 118
Mexico Declaration (2000), 14
Meyer, G. and Dearing, J., 134
micro-environmental factors, as health
    determinants, 8, 9
migrants, 92–4
Milio, N., 6, 22, 23
Millar, B., 157
Mind Out programme, 87
Minkler, M., 56
Moos, R. and Schaefer, J., 66
mortality rates, 7
    infant, 26, 95
    in Ireland, 10, 26
    socioeconomic status, 10, 65
    Travelling community, 95
multiculturalism, 91–6
Murray, C. and Lopez, A., 89
Myross Community Development Network, 54

Naidoo, J. and Wills, J., 56
*National Action Plan against Poverty and Social
    Exclusion 2003–2005*, 19

national agreements, 19, 24
National Economic and Social Council (NESC), 23
National Health Promotion Strategy (2000), 16, 17, 57, 90
National Health Promotion Strategy (2002–2005), 79
National Public Speaking Project, 87
natural science, 109, 110
naturalistic research, 109, 111–12
Needs and Abilities report, 28
needs assessment, 45
needs, normative, 45
Newman Giger, J. and Davidhizar, R., 93
Nightingale, Florence, 78, 80
Nolan, B., 10
non-maleficence, 141
normative needs, 45
North–South Ireland Food Consumption Survey, 60
Nuremberg Code of Ethics, 139
nurses, and health-promotion, 78–84
  attitudes and understanding, 79–81
  barriers and challenges, 80–1
  confusion with health education, 79, 80, 81
  definitions of nursing, 78
  empowering nurses, 81–3
  in Ireland, 81
  lifestyles of nurses, 83–4
  models of nursing, 13–14, 78, 80
  political involvement, 82
  role models, 79, 83–4
  smoking by nurses, 84, 97
  work–life balance, 63
Nutbeam, D. and Harris, E., 41, 44
nutrition, 60

obesity, 60
  exercise and, 57
  mental illness and, 96
objectives, 'SMART', 46, 173
occupational health units, 71
occupational stress, 61, 66–7
  management, 71
OECD (Organisation for Economic Co-operation and Development), 26
On My Own Two Feet programme, 77
opinion leaders, 44, 46
organisation, culture of, 68–70
organisation, definition of, 67
organisational change, 42–7
  diffusion of innovations theory, 44
  evaluation, 46–7
  force field analysis, 43

Lewin's unfreezing/freezing model, 42–3
  stages of, 44–7
Ottawa Charter (1986), 12–13, 81, 133
  definition of health, 12
  definition of health promotion, 13
  empowerment, 48, 53, 114
  framework for health promotion, 18
  planning and development, 21–2, 44
  'settings approach', 70
  social capital promotion, 53
Out and About Association, 88
outcome evaluation, 46, 135

Papandopoulos, I., 93
Parahoo, K., 140, 142
parental leave, 64
Park Dorsay, J. and Forchuk, C., 98
Patton, D. *et al.*, 98
Paul Partnership, 54
Peplau, H., 79
personal factors, as health determinants, 7–9, 10
phenomenology, 116–22
  intentionality of consciousness, 117–18
  intuiting, 117, 118
  lived experience/life-world, 118, 119–20
  reduction, 118–19
  role of researcher, 120–2
physical activity, 56–8
  barriers/motivators, 57
Piper, S. and Brown, P., 82
planned behaviour theory, 37
planning, 21–3, 28–30
  action planning, 44–5
  action research and, 129
  contingency planning, 29
  good planning, 28–9
    trategic management, 30
policy *see* public policy
politics
  political factors and health, 9
  public policy and, 31–3
Poor Law Unions, 24–5
positivism, 105, 108, 109, 117–18, 166
  positivist research, 110–11
postpositivism, 111
post-test design, 135
poverty, 9, 10, 24, 65, 85, 86
Powell, J., 136
power, 14, 50–2, 74
  critical theory and elitism, 113–15
  disempowerment, 50, 113–15
  expert power, 50–1
  in organisations, 68, 69
  types of, 50

power, *continued*
  unethical research and, 139, 142, 143
  see also empowerment
pre-test design, 135
preventative services, 9
primary healthcare, 12
privacy, right to, 144
probability sampling, 168
process evaluation, 46, 134–5
Prochaska, J., 37
  and DiClemente, C., 38
Programme for Prosperity and Fairness, 63
Programme for the Disabled, 27
Promoting Health/Preventing Disease: Objectives for the Nation, 12
Promoting Increased Physical Activity, 57–8
proposals, research, 173–7
Prospectus Report (2003), 28
Psychiatric Programme, 27
psychiatric services, 85, 88–90, 96
  objectives of, 89
  see also mental health promotion; mental illness
Psychiatric Services: Planning for the Future, 28, 88
psychological functioning, and health, 3, 4
psychology, 74–5
public policy, 5, 16–20, 21–33
  expenditure, 24, 26, 27
  globalisation, effects of, 27–8
  'healthy public policy', 20, 23, 31–2, 74
  historical, 24–6, 28, 30
  influences on, 3–5, 18, 33
  national health strategies, 16–20
  planning and strategy, 21–3, 28–30
  politics, 31–3
  shifting of responsibility, 56
  social policy, 23–6, 74
purposive sampling, 168
Putnam, R., 52

Quality and Fairness: A Health System for You, 17–18, 90, 91, 99
questionnaires, 137, 166–7, 169–71, 175
  types of questions, 169–70
  see also surveys
questions, open and closed, 160, 169
quota sampling, 168

Ramos, M., 84
random selection, 168–9
randomised control trials (RCTs), 105, 150
Rappaport, J., Swift, C. and Hess, R., 49
reasoned action theory, 37

reciprocal determinism, 41
reduction, phenomenological, 118–19
reductionism, 84, 87–8, 106
reflective practice, 134–5
refugees, 92
Reid, A. and Malone, J., 71
Relationships and Sexuality Education (RSE), 76, 77, 87
relativism, 140
research, 108–12
  action research, 47, 126–32
  bias, 170
  critical theory, 114–15, 126
  empirical, 105, 110–11, 123
  ethics, 139–45
    research contracts, 144
  evaluation, 133–8
  evidence-based practice, 105–7
  experiments, 105, 110, 119
  grounded theory, 123–5
  inductive, 123
  interviews, 151–6
  literature reviews, 146–50
  naturalistic research, 109, 111–12
  objective and rationale, 173–4
  paradigms, 108–12, 174
  phenomenology, 116–22
  positivist research, 110–11
  qualitative, 108, 111, 151, 157, 163
  quantitative, 108, 128, 137
  research approach and methods, 108, 173–7
  rights of participants, 142–5
  surveys, 165–72
  validation, 130–1
  writing a proposal, 173–7
respect
  for autonomy (principle of respect), 141–2
  right to respect, 142–3
rights, 140, 142–5
  Universal Declaration of Human Rights, 31–2, 92, 104
  see also ethics
Robinson, N., 157
Rodin, J. and Salovey, P., 66
Rogers, E., 44
Rosenstock, L., 36
Rowe, K. and Macleod Clark, J., 79
Royal College of Nursing, 98
RSE (Relationships and Sexuality Education), 76, 77, 87
Rush, K. *et al.*, 83, 84

Sackett, D. *et al.*, 103
Sadala, M. and de Camargo Ferreira Adorno, R.,

117, 118
safety at work, 66, 70–1
Safety, Health and Welfare at Work Act 1989, 71
sampling, 168–9
    focus group selection, 159–60
    probability/non-probability, 137, 168
    random selection, 168–9
    in surveys, 167–9
    theoretical sampling, 125
    types of, 168–9
Sartre, Jean Paul, 117
Schein, E., 68, 69
schizophrenia, 97–8 see also mental illness
Schizophrenia Ireland, 88
schools see education, health promotion in
science, 109
scientific knowledge, 105, 108, 109
self-determination, 141–2, 144
self-efficacy, 35, 36, 41, 51
self-esteem, 35, 75, 85, 86, 90
Senior, B., 68
sexual education, 76, 77
sexual health, 60
    and mental illness, 98–9
Shaping a Healthier Future, 16, 17, 30, 57, 79, 95
sickness, concept of, 2 see also illness
SIDS (sudden infant death syndrome), 95
Simons-Morton, B., Green, W. and Gottlieb, N., 7
Sines, D., 83
Skinner, 80
SLÁN (Survey of Lifestyles, Attitudes and Nutrition), 10, 58, 59
Slí na Sláinte, 58
SMART objectives, 46, 173
smoking, 58–9
    ban, 26, 41, 58–9, 72
        exemption, 97
    by nurses, 84, 97
    example of health promoter role, 56
    mental illness and, 97–8
    statistics, 26, 58–9
snowball sampling, 168
Social and Personal Health Education (SPHE), 76, 77, 87
social capital, 52–3
social class, and health, 9, 10, 65
social cognition theory, 40–2, 44, 75, 84
social environment, as health determinant, 7–9, 10, 41, 55, 56
social inequality, 9, 10, 65, 74, 113
social isolation, 85, 86
social justice, 49, 51

social learning theory, 40–2, 44, 75, 84
social partnership, 19, 24
social policy, 23–6, 74
social realism, 124
social science, 109, 110, 111
social services, 24
socialisation, 41
socioeconomic status, and health, 9, 10, 65
sociology, 73–4
sociopolitical factors, and health, 8, 9, 10, 14
Solutions for Wellness programme, 96
SPHE (Social and Personal Health Education), 76, 77, 87
Spielberg, H., 116
spirituality, 4, 84
sports, 57
Spring, B. et al., 97
stages of change model, 37–40, 75, 80
Statistical Package for the Social Sciences (SPSS), 175
Stay Safe Programme, 77
Stenhouse, Lawrence, 128, 131
Stevens, P., 164
Stewart, D. and Shamdasani, P., 159, 161, 162
STIs (sexually transmitted infections), 60
Stone, G. et al., 66
strategic management, 30 see also planning
Strauss, A., 123–4
    and Corbin, J., 124
stress, 35, 85, 86, 87
    management, 71
    work-related, 61, 66–7, 71
Stumpf, Carl, 116–17
subjective norms, 37
subjectivity, 119
sudden infant death syndrome (SIDS), 95
suicide, 85, 86, 87
    rates in Ireland, 89
summative evaluation, 135
Survey of Lifestyles, Attitudes and Nutrition (SLÁN), 10, 58, 59
surveys, 165–72
    bias in, 170
    data analysis, 171–2
    data collection methods, 166–71
    sampling in, 167–9
    types of questions, 169–70
    validity and reliability, 170–1
sustainability, 13
Sustaining Progress 2003–2005, 19
SWOT analysis, 46

tape-recording, in research, 154, 161, 163
Taylor, L., 86

Taylor, M., 104
Than, M. *et al.*, 104
theoretical sampling, 125
theory of reasoned action (planned behaviour),
   37
Thomas, Karen, 42
Thorogood, N., 73
Tones, K., 23
   and Green, G., 14, 15, 23, 36, 50, 53, 70
Torre, D., 49
*Towards better Healthcare Management in the
   Health Board*, 25
transtheoretical model of change, 37–40
Travelling community, 94–6
Tuskagee study, 139

unemployment, 65, 85, 86
unfreezing/freezing model of change, 42–3
United Nations, 33
   Universal Declaration of Human Rights, 31–2,
      92, 104
Upshur, R., 105
Usher, P., 114
utilitarian philosophy, 140

validation, 130–1
vicarious learning, 41, 44
victim blaming, 56

Waar, P., 66
Walk Tall programme, 77
Walker, K., 103
Wallerstein, N., 49
Warr, P., 66
Weisberg, H. *et al.*, 165, 166
welfare system, 3, 65
wellbeing, 2, 4, 6–7, 13, 48
   empowerment and, 48
   exercise and, 56
   mental health, 85, 87, 88
   work environment and, 65, 66–7

Whitehead, D., 14, 80, 81
Whitehead, J., 128–9
WHO *see* World Health Organization
'wholeness', 2 *see also* holistic concept of health
Wiley, M., 24, 26
Wilson, G., 35
Winter, R. and Munn-Giddings, C., 128, 131,
   132
Woodrow, P., 82
work, 61–72
   health and work, 61, 65–7
   health promotion in workplace, 70–2
      Ireland, 63, 64, 72
   importance of, 63, 65, 66
   job flexibility, 63, 64
   organisation culture and structure, 67–70
   safety at work, 66, 70–1
   supportive supervisors, 66
   work–life balance, 61–4
      conflict, 61
workhouses, 24
Work–Life Balance Day, 63
World Bank, 33
World Federation for Mental Health, 89
World Health Organization (WHO), 2, 3–5, 33
   defining health, 3–5
   empowerment promotion, 53, 83, 134
   'Health for all by the year 2000' (1978), 12
   healthy public policy, 31
   mental health promotion, 89
   principles of health promotion, 18, 75, 115
   schools initiative, 78
   see also Ottawa Charter
World Psychiatric Association, 89
Wren, Barbara, 42
writing a research proposal, 173–7
Wynne, R., 71

The Years Ahead report, 28
Yuro-Petro, H. and Scanelli, B., 83